Acquisition and Performance of Sports Skills

Terry McMorris
University College, Chichester, UK

John Wiley & Sons, Ltd

This publication is designed to provide accurate and authoritative information in regard to
the subject matter covered. It is sold on the understanding that the Publisher is not engaged
in rendering professional services. If professional advice or other expert assistance is
required, the services of a competent professional should be sought.

Other Wiley Editorial Offices

John Wiley & Sons Inc., 111 River Street, Hoboken, NJ 07030, USA

Jossey-Bass, 989 Market Street, San Francisco, CA 94103-1741, USA

Wiley-VCH Verlag GmbH, Boschstr. 12, D-69469 Weinheim, Germany

John Wiley & Sons Australia Ltd, 33 Park Road, Milton, Queensland 4064, Australia

John Wiley & Sons (Asia) Pte Ltd, 2 Clementi Loop #02-01, Jin Xing Distripark, Singapore
129809

John Wiley & Sons Canada Ltd, 22 Worcester Road, Etobicoke, Ontario, Canada
M9W 1L1

Wiley also publishes its books in a variety of electronic formats. Some content that appears
in print may not be available in electronic books.

Library of Congress Cataloging-in-Publication Data

McMorris, Terry.
Acquisition and performance of sports skills / Terry McMorris.
    p.   cm. – (Wiley SportTexts)
    Includes bibliographical references and index.
    ISBN 0-470-84994-0 (cloth : alk. paper) – ISBN 0-470-84995-9 (pbk. : alk. paper)
    1. Sports sciences.   2. Sports–Psychological aspects.   3. Athletic ability.   I. Title.
    II. Series.
GV558.M36   2004
796.01–dc22   2004000843

British Library Cataloguing in Publication Data

A catalogue record for this book is available from the British Library

ISBN: 978-0-470-84995-8 (P/B)
ISBN: 978-0-470-84994-1 (H/B)

Typeset in 11/14pt Sabon by Keytec Typesetting Ltd, Bridport, Dorset
Printed and bound in Great Britain by CPI Antony Rowe, Chippenham, Wilts

Contents

Acquisition and Performance of Sports Skills   T. McMorris
© 2004 John Wiley & Sons, Ltd   ISBNs: 0-470-84994-0 (HB); 0-470-84995-9 (PB)

Series Preface

One of the most astonishing cultural phenomena of the twentieth century has been the exponential growth in our knowledge and understanding of the importance of sport and exercise to human kind. At the beginning of that century, sport was principally a force for moral development, whilst strenuous exercise, though necessary to ensure military personnel were fit to engage in combat, was medically prescribed. The academic study of sport – what there was of it – was restricted largely to the history of the Olympic Games and philosophical arguments for the moral case for team games. A hundred years later, the picture is very different. Four hundred million people turn on their television sets to watch the Opening Ceremony of the Olympic Games and soccer's World Cup Final; millions of people jog, go to the gym, or work out in front of the television; and the academic study of sport embraces physics, chemistry, biology, biomechanics, physiology, psychology, politics, sociology, social anthropology and business studies, as well as history and philosophy. Over the last 20 years the number of degree courses in the academic study of sport and exercise has grown phenomenally, attracting students from a wide range of backgrounds. It is against this background that the new series *Wiley SportTexts* was conceived.

This new series provides a collection of textbooks in Sport and Exercise Science that is rooted in the student's practical experience of sport. Each book covers the theoretical foundations of the contributing disciplines from the natural, human, behavioural and social sciences, and provides the theoretical, practical and conceptual tools needed for the rigorous academic study of sport. Individual texts focus on a specific learning stage from the various levels of undergraduate to postgraduate study.

The series adopts a student-centred, interactive, problem-solving approach to key issues, and encourages the student to develop autonomous learning strategies through self-assessment exercises. Each chapter begins with clear learning

Acquisition and Performance of Sports Skills   T. McMorris
© 2004 John Wiley & Sons, Ltd   ISBNs: 0-470-84994-0 (HB); 0-470-84995-9 (PB)

objectives and a concise summary of the key concepts covered. A glossary of important terms and symbols familiarizes students with the language and conventions of the various academic communities studying sport. Worked examples and solutions to exercises, together with a variety of formative and summative self-assessment tasks, are also included, supported by key references in book, journal and electronic forms. The series will also have a dedicated website with specific information on individual titles, supplementary information for lecturers, important developments in the academic study of sport, and links to other sites of interest.

It is intended that the series will eventually provide a complete coverage of the mainstream elements of taught undergraduate and postgraduate degrees in the study of sport.

Tudor Hale, Jim Parry and **Roger Bartlett**
April 2003

Prologue

To those of us interested in sport, skilful performances bring a great deal of pleasure, whether it is our own performance of a skill or observing others perform. For most people, I think that their own performance is more important, even if the level is not particularly high. Our efforts may not be seen by many other people but, nevertheless, they still please us. Some individuals reach the top of their sport, and their performances thrill not only themselves but also millions of spectators around the world. Generally, we most readily appreciate the performance of skills in our own sport. However, observation of great performances in other activities can also be exciting; even though our knowledge of the sport may be limited we 'just know' that what we are watching is of a high quality.

It is fitting that I am writing this Prologue on the anniversary of one of the most famous tries ever scored in Rugby Union – Gareth Edwards' try for the Barbarians against the New Zealand All Blacks in 1973. Although Rugby is not my game and my knowledge of it is limited, I still enjoy watching that try – from the initial individual brilliance of Phil Bennett, through the inter-passing of many of the team, to the finish by Edwards. Another demonstration of skill that was a pleasure to watch was an ice dance performance by Jayne Torvill and Christopher Dean, which I saw on television in 1985. I cannot skate, and I do not particularly like ice dance, but the quality was such that even I could enjoy their remarkable skill.

Another perspective on watching skilled performances is that of a coach. Seeing someone perform a skill that you have taught them is a most rewarding experience, especially if it was the result of a great deal of hard work. This book examines what is happening, mentally and neuropsychologically, when we perform skills and how we are able to acquire such skills. The study of these phenomena has made me more appreciative of top-class performances and I hope that it also helps you to enjoy playing, spectating and/or coaching even more than you do at present.

Acquisition and Performance of Sports Skills   T. McMorris
© 2004 John Wiley & Sons, Ltd   ISBNs: 0-470-84994-0 (HB); 0-470-84995-9 (PB)

This book is designed primarily for those of you embarking on the study of the acquisition and performance of sports skills at degree level. Parts of it will also be useful to those who have passed the beginner stage. I hope, however, that it might also be of interest to those who are not formally studying the subject but who have an interest in it whether as a player, a coach or a spectator. Since the book is aimed primarily at students, it follows the basic format of a textbook. Each chapter begins with a brief outline of the learning objectives for the chapter. At the end of each chapter, there are key points in note form, which I hope will help students with revision. Also, there are questions and problems which will test your understanding and help prepare you for formal examinations. I have used a variety of methods of testing; many you will have come across previously but some may be new to you. At the end of each chapter, I have listed books and/or journal articles which I recommend you to read. Some of these are at the same level as this book, while others take the study of a particular topic further.

Within the text, I have occasionally suggested that you try some things out for yourself. Although I guess that many of you will not be inclined to do this, I strongly urge you to do so because these little activities are designed to help your understanding of the acquisition and performance of skills. I would also encourage you to take time to think about your own experiences and examine to what extent they can be explained by the theories and research covered in this book. Similarly, it is a good idea to talk to other people about their experiences, especially if their backgrounds in sport differ from yours.

This book is part of a series, published by John Wiley and Sons Ltd, and as such will follow the same format as the other books in the series. The idea is to write a 'user friendly' text. Many students find the academic style of writing used in many textbooks, even those for beginners, very daunting. Therefore, the books in this series are written in more accessible English. Similarly, we have deliberately refrained from excessive citation of authors. Constantly citing authors is off-putting to beginners and can make the text difficult to read. Despite this I am well aware that, as you develop your knowledge base and become more experienced, you will be expected to write in a more academic style. There are several styles which are accepted by sports psychologists. The most commonly used is that described in the *Publication Manual of the American Psychology Association* (American Psychology Association, 2002). Those of you who are at University should consult with your own tutors and examine your institution's guidelines to see what style they recommend. In Appendix 1, I have written a short passage in the style I have used in this book; I have then re-written the passage using APA style. Perhaps the most important factor for you to note is that, in a formal academic style, you must cite authors to support your claims. You cannot, as I have done in this text, simply state 'research has shown'; you need to say which research.

Almost all introductory texts on the acquisition and performance of sports skills follow an Information Processing Theory approach. Although other theories have been known for some time, this theory has had the greatest following. Recently, however, a large number of sports psychologists have moved their allegiance to what we term ecological psychology theories. Until very recently, I always took an Information Processing Theory approach with my first- and second-level students and only introduced ecological theories at the third level. I have changed this in the last few years for two important reasons. First of all, it is becoming impossible to read journals and more advanced texts without finding references to ecological theories. Secondly, and more importantly, I have found that by introducing ecological theories at an earlier stage students are able to perceive the strengths and weaknesses of each of the schools of thought rather than becoming comfortable with one idea and then having to rethink their whole position. Many students have said to me that learning Information Processing Theory first and then ecological theories was something like watching two party-political broadcasts; after the first one you are convinced that party is correct, but change your mind following the second broadcast. By covering both schools of thought at the same time we can overcome this problem. Obviously you may choose to concentrate on one theory and skip the other. Similarly, tutors can recommend the use of all of the text or advise their students to concentrate on certain areas.

Although to some extent the theories are opposed, in fact that is not always the case. Information Processing Theory is based on a cognitive approach to explain our actions. Ecological psychology theorists are not interested in cognition; they are more concerned with explaining performance from what we can actually see. Ecological psychologists like to talk about what we observe directly, while Information Processing theorists prefer to take what we see as the first step in explaining what is happening in our brain. Due to the fact that the two theories differ in their fundamental approaches, sometimes they are complementary, other times they are diametrically opposed and sometimes the explanations of action are simply from different perspectives.

I have tried, in this text, to be as neutral as possible when covering each theory. In fact, like many other sports psychologists, I favour some form of hybrid theory that combines the best of both schools of thought. However, we need a great deal more research before any of us can devise a theory that totally explains how we perform and acquire skills. This latter point leads me to another aspect of the study of skill acquisition and performance, and indeed the study of almost all sports science. There are very few definitive answers. Most phenomena can only be partially explained. There is a great deal that cannot be fully understood at this moment in time. To some students this is galling as they expect answers, but to others it is exciting. You could be the person who explains some phenomenon which has puzzled scientists for years. While this is probably unlikely, the chance of increasing knowledge about a topic just a small amount is not as remote as you might think. As you progress through your studies, the opportunity to carry out research projects occurs. These will not be great Nobel Prize-winning studies but may still advance our knowledge. Some of my past undergraduate students have carried out research projects which have subsequently been published in academic journals. You too could achieve that distinction. Many of you will not aspire to publications but simply want to increase your own knowledge base. Whatever your reasons for reading this book, I hope that you will get even half as much pleasure from studying skills as I do; but I must admit that studying them does not beat actually performing the skills.

Terry McMorris

1 Skill, Ability and Performance

Learning Objectives

By the end of this chapter, you should be able to

♦ understand what is meant by the term 'skill'

　◇ be able to place skills into categories

　◇ be able to analyse the factors underlying skilled performance

　◇ understand what is meant by the term abilities

　◇ understand the theories of ability

♦ understand the skill–ability interaction

♦ understand the basics of Information Processing Theory

♦ understand the basics of ecological psychology (Action Systems and Dynamical Systems) theories

Acquisition and Performance of Sports Skills　T. McMorris
© 2004 John Wiley & Sons, Ltd　ISBNs: 0-470-84994-0 (HB); 0-470-84995-9 (PB)

Introduction

In the first part of this chapter, we examine what is meant by the term 'skill' and how we divide skills into different classifications. The reader is urged to consider the efficacy of these classifications and to question the value of their usage. The second part of the chapter examines ability. The use of the word ability can be misleading. Its use in everyday language compared to its usage in psychology can cause some confusion. Moreover, the reader may wish to question the whole concept of abilities, as defined by psychologists. In the third part of the chapter, we examine the inter-relationship between skill and ability. Finally, the chapter concludes with overviews of Information Processing Theory and the ecological psychology theories of skilled performance.

The basis of the explanations of skill and ability used in this chapter are found in Information Processing Theory. Some references to ecological theories are made. However, in general, ecological psychologists tend to use terms such as action and movement to describe skill. They are not concerned about classifications as such. They are interested in how the person's genetic make-up affects their performance, but have little interest in trying to put labels on these factors.

Skill

There are many definitions concerning what we mean by skill. Fortunately most have several common features. It is generally accepted that skill is *learned*, *consistent* and *specific* to the task. Moreover, it is *goal oriented*, i.e., the person is aiming to achieve some specific outcome. This outcome can be quantitative, determined by the performance of a movement that can be measured objectively; or qualitative, measured by subjective judgement. Therefore, in this book we will use the following working definition of skill: *skill is the consistent production of goal-oriented movements, which are learned and specific to the task.*

In order to examine the nature of skill further, we can focus on each of the components of our working definition, one at a time. Firstly, skills are learned rather than innate. Although we often hear people say that someone is a 'born' footballer or tennis player, this is not correct. Even the very basic skills, such as walking, running, striking and jumping, need to be learned. Subsequent skills that we acquire, such as catching a ball, doing a somersault or hitting a tennis ball, are refinements of the basic skills and need to be learned. Moreover, we cannot say that we have acquired a skill until we can perform it consistently. We have all seen examples of 'beginner's luck'. The first time that I ever set foot on a putting green, at the age of seven, I holed a 10 m putt. Unfortunately dreams of fame and fortune as a tournament golfer quickly evaporated at the next hole, where I took more hits than Tiger Woods takes to get round all 18 holes.

While I doubt that anyone would question the fact that we cannot say that we have acquired a skill until we can perform it consistently, I think that some readers may have difficulty in accepting that a skill must be learned. I know that many of my students have problems with this concept. It is my belief that the difficulty arises due to what we mean by learning. To most people learning a skill is explicit, i.e., we consciously set out to perform something that we have seen or are told to do. If this were the case, we could not argue that skills must be learned, as we acquire many skills without consciously trying to copy someone or follow a set of instructions. This is particularly so in childhood, when we develop our basic skills. Learning can occur implicitly or sub-consciously. We often acquire skills without instruction, by simply setting out to achieve a goal. This can be seen when babies learn to crawl in order to reach an object that they wish to touch. They have received no instruction but still manage to crawl. Implicit learning, however, does not only take place in early childhood, it can happen any time when we set out to achieve a goal (see Chapter 8). The key factor is that we can only achieve the goal by learning to carry out the movement.

Whether we learn a skill explicitly or implicitly, the skill is specific to the goal we are trying to achieve. In other words, each skill is unique. That does not mean that there will not be similarities between skills or that the ability to perform one skill will not make the acquisition of another skill easier. The uniqueness of skills can be seen by comparing skills that are very similar to one another. As an example, I will use the lofted pass and chip pass in soccer. Both are struck with the same part of the foot and in both instances the ball needs to be struck beneath the mid-point. In order to go in a straight line, it needs to be kicked along the central axis. For the lofted pass, however, the striker must follow through after contact. For the chip, there is very little follow through and the point of foot–ball contact is much nearer to the bottom of the ball. The uniqueness of the two skills can be seen by the fact that soccer players who are good at performing one of the skills are not necessarily good at performing the other. However, many are good at both skills.

Think of some examples of similar skills from your own sport and list the similarities and differences. See if you can think of any skills that are identical. I doubt very much that you can. Even running with a Rugby ball in your hands is different to running freely. Running while dribbling a hockey ball is very different from free running or even just running while carrying a hockey stick, without having to dribble the ball.

In the previous two paragraphs, we introduced the notion that skill is a goal-oriented activity. The nature of the goal will determine the way in which we evaluate the level of its performance. The goal of many skills is to perform some act that is measured solely by a quantitative outcome. Examples of this are activities like running the 100 m, throwing a javelin and passing a netball to a teammate. Performance of such skills can be objectively measured. The running of 100 m can be measured in time or by competition against other runners, the javelin by how far you throw and the netball pass by the accuracy. In such skills it is the *outcome* that is crucial, not how you look while performing the skill. In lay language, skill to perform such tasks often gets mixed up with how one looks while performing the skill. Psychologists call the latter *form*. Form, however, is not the important factor in such skills but outcome is. It is true that many skilful performers, whose outcome is very good, also demonstrate good form. We can all think of performers who look graceful. When I think of sprinters, who exhibit good form, I think of Maurice Greene. However, when I think of great sprinters, I also think of Michael Johnson. Johnson's style would not be shown in a coaching manual but he is one of the greatest sprinters of all time.

I could go on and on giving examples of performers who demonstrate good form and good outcome and athletes whose style does not follow the coaching manual or which is not aesthetically pleasing. The way in which each person achieves a particular goal will differ due to their individual make-up. Biomechanists will tell you that very few people, if any, are capable of performing in the way in which biomechanical models of the correct performance suggest. This is because biomechanical models are based on the assumption that the individual possesses a normal range of movement, normal bone structure and so on. Very few of us are totally 'normal' physically. There are very few people who are totally symmetrical, for example. Individual differences will result in people performing the same skill in very different ways.

While a lack of style is acceptable for a skill in which the measurement is an outcome, a breakaway from the accepted norm, when performing, would be unsuitable for a skill that is subjectively measured on the basis of its aesthetic appeal. Such qualitative skills are found in gymnastics, dance and ice-skating. In these skills, form is the measurement of skilfulness rather than outcome.

Classification of skills

In the previous section, we highlighted the fact that skill is goal oriented. As a result, many psychologists think that, rather than classifying skills, we should simply state the goal of a skill and not try to place it into a specific category, along with other skills. While I tend to agree with this line of thought, I think that it is important that we examine the attempts to classify skills for two reasons. Firstly, the classifications used are a good introduction to the analysis of specific skills. Secondly, you will come across these classifications in your reading, therefore you need to know to what the writers are referring.

The first classification of skill that I will cover is *fine motor* versus *gross motor* skills. Fine motor skills are rarely, if ever, found in sport and are skills which require the use of few limbs and are undertaken in limited space, e.g., writing, typing and sewing. On the other hand, most sports skills are gross motor skills. They require the use of several limbs, often the whole body, and tend to take place in a comparatively large amount of space. Despite the fact that sports skills are gross motor skills, much that has been written about skill acquisition comes from research using fine motor skills. Although the American Information Processing Theorist Robert Singer pointed this anomaly out in the 1960s (Singer, 1968), it is only recently that researchers have begun to examine gross motor skills. It is particularly sobering to realize that much of what we teach coaches and physical education teachers, concerning the teaching and learning of sports skills, is based on research with fine motor skills.

Whether fine or gross, skills have been divided into *discrete*, *serial* and *continuous*. Discrete skills are those with a definable beginning and end, such as a set shot in basketball, a free-kick in soccer or a throw in any sport. Discrete skills concern the performance of *one* action in isolation from other actions. On the other hand, serial skills are when we join together two or more discrete skills, e.g., the triple jump. Like discrete skills, they have a definite beginning and end but one component leads into another. So, in the triple jump, the hop leads to the step which leads to the jump. Many gymnastics movements, particularly in floor exercises, are examples of serial skills. On the other hand, continuous skills have no recognizable beginning or end. The person can start or stop when they choose. Examples of continuous skills are running, walking, paddling a canoe and swimming. This classification can be useful to us when examining some aspects of practice and learning.

One of the most used classifications of skill, and one which you will definitely come across in your reading, is *simple* versus *complex* skills. To me, this is the most controversial of the classifications. The notion of simple and complex skills, as used in the motor learning literature, is based on cognitive theories.

This is reflected by the fact that simple skills are said to be those which require little in the way of information processing demands, while complex skills involve much information processing. Simple skills, therefore, would include hitting a golf ball or carrying out a gymnastics routine, where there is little in the nature of decision making and the emphasis is on technique. On the other hand, complex skills would be skills such as passing a basketball. In such a skill, the main factor is not the technical difficulty but the decision of where and when to pass the ball. To call the former skill simple is, in my opinion, to underestimate the neuropsychological demands. Try telling a golfer that it is simple to hit a golf ball accurately!

However, there is definitely a difference in the demands of skills that require little in the nature of decision making compared with those that require much. Where little information processing is required, technique is the key factor. Where decision making is important, it is the choice of which technique to use in any given situation that is the major issue. The British psychologist Poulton (1957) did not use the terms simple and complex, but rather *open* and *closed*, to distinguish between these kinds of skills. According to Poulton, open skills require much in the way of information processing and take place in environments that are rarely, if ever, completely repeated. The change in environment means that every time the skill is performed, the performer must modify his/her technique to achieve the same goal, or even use a different technique to achieve the goal. Closed skills, on the other hand, take place in the same or very similar environments, therefore the same technique can be used over and over again. Poulton, however, was aware that you could not simply divide skills into *two* categories. Therefore, he claimed that the open–closed classification was best described as being a continuum. Most sports skills will fall nearer to the open end of the continuum than to the closed, although the shot putt is a good example of a closed skill. The size and weight of the shot, the target area and the size of the circle do not alter from one putt to another.

Ann Gentile and colleagues (Gentile *et al.*, 1975) refined Poulton's classification by trying to give some examples of the differences between closed and open situations. The classification does try to take into account some of the neuropsychological differences in tasks, but is still heavily biased towards the importance of decision making and information processing (Figure 1.1).

It is up to readers to decide for themselves how much they like or dislike the idea of classifying skills, and indeed which type of classification they prefer. Before leaving the subject, however, we need to evaluate whether it is better simply to break down the skill into its component parts rather than placing it into a definitive category. By breaking down a skill, I mean that we should examine the neuropsychological, perceptual and decision-making demands of the skill.

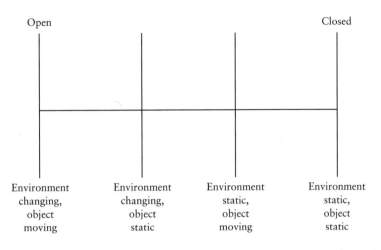

Figure 1.1 Diagrammatic representation of Gentile *et al.*'s (1975) open–closed skill classification

The advantage of breaking down a skill is that you deal with the *specific* skill rather than a generalized concept, e.g., open or closed. Also, you are less likely to focus just on the cognitive aspects of the skill to the detriment of the neuropsychological demands. According to Poulton's classification, making a pass with the inside of the foot, in a soccer game, falls well towards the open end of the continuum. Similarly, passing the ball with the outside of the foot and making it swerve also falls close to the open end of the continuum. However, the neuropsychological demands are far greater in the latter, therefore it is a more difficult skill to perform.

Breaking a skill down into its component parts is not as simple as it may seem. Here I will present a breakdown of catching a ball. I will keep it as simple as possible and we will return to it later in the chapter. In order to catch a ball the person must first judge the line and length of flight. They must determine the speed at which the ball is travelling. Then they need to move their hands into the line of flight. They have to decide what style of catch to use, one hand or two, fingers pointing up or down. Immediately prior to hand-ball contact they must 'give', so that the ball does not rebound from a solid surface. They, also, have to close their fingers around the ball at precisely the correct moment. Just a simple skill!

Ability

The word ability is used in everyday language to describe either the skills we possess or how well we can perform a skill. We may say that someone has the ability to perform a particular task or that another person has great ability in a particular activity. The word ability is used in psychology in exactly the same way, but it is also used in psychology to describe *basic innate actions that underlie skilful performance*. It is easy to confuse these abilities with basic skills, such as walking, running, jumping and so on. However, as we have seen those skills are learned, while abilities are innate. Moreover, the amount of and types of abilities that we possess are determined genetically. We naturally acquire these abilities as we develop, although they can be improved by practice. The amount of improvement, however, is limited by genetic factors. It is generally thought that it is the amount and type of abilities that we possess that underpin our proficiency in particular skills. Thus, one person has the necessary abilities to become a gymnast, while another may possess the abilities necessary to become a good Rugby player.

The idea that we possess innate abilities that underlie our ability to acquire and perform sports skills has been with us for some time. This basic premise has, until very recently, gone unchallenged. More recently, Ericsson and co-workers (e.g., Ericsson, Krampe and Teschromer 1993) have claimed that everyone has the ability to perform *all* skills, if they practice sufficiently. This claim is directly opposed to the notion of abilities underlying skilful perform-ance and the genetic nature of abilities.

The notion that we are born with certain natural abilities has intuitive appeal. We only have to observe the people around us to see that different individuals possess different talents. We all know people that 'have an ear for music' or are good at skills that require the use of their hands. The idea that people have abilities that predispose them to acquiring many skills in sport led to the notion of a 'born' sports person. It was said that such people possess what is called *general motor ability*. Anecdotal evidence supports this claim. Many individuals appear to be good at whatever sport they take up. However, empirical evidence from research tends not to support this claim.

The major researchers into motor ability have been the Americans Franklin Henry (1968) and Edwin Fleishman (1954, 1967). Henry undertook his research with students at the University of California at Berkeley, USA, while Fleishman's research was with American military personnel. Both researchers undertook huge studies examining the abilities possessed by hundreds of people. After carrying out statistical analyses on the data, they both came to the conclusion that there was no such thing as general motor ability. Henry found no evidence of any significant relationships between the abilities he examined. He therefore decided that abilities were *specific* and *unique*. Henry explained the 'born' sports person by saying that there were people who possess many specific abilities, therefore they would give the impression of possessing general motor ability. Unlike Henry, Fleishman showed that some abilities were correlated, albeit moderately at best, and could be clustered into groups. The abilities that were related tended to be ones that we might expect, e.g., static balance, dynamic balance and ballistic balance. Fleishman's theory is known as the *factor analysis hypothesis*, because factor analysis is the statistical procedure he used to determine his clusters. Table 1.1 outlines the clusters identified by Fleishman.

In teaching the nature of ability over a period of more years than I care to remember, I have found very few students who readily accept the findings of Henry and Fleishman. There is a great deal of anecdotal evidence to suggest

Table 1.1 Fleishman's ability clusters (based on Fleishman, 1967)

Psychomotor factors	Physical factors
1. Control precision (control over fast, accurate movements that use large areas of the body)	1. Extent (or static) flexibility
2. Multilimb co-ordination	2. Dynamic flexibility
3. Response orientation (selection of the appropriate response)	3. Static strength
4. Reaction time	4. Dynamic strength
5. Speed of arm movement	5. Explosive strength
6. Rate control (coincidence-anticipation)	6. Trunk strength
7. Manual dexterity	7. Gross body co-ordination
8. Arm–hand steadiness	8. Gross body equilibrium
9. Wrist–finger speed (co-ordination of fast wrist and finger movements)	9. Stamina (cardiovascular fitness)
10. Aiming	
11. Postural discrimination (co-ordination when vision is occluded)	
12. Response integration (integration of sensory information to produce a movement)	

that there *is* such a thing as general motor ability. We cannot, however, simply write off the findings of Henry and Fleishman. Their research had very large sample sizes and was carried out over a period of many years. One explanation for the anomaly between the research findings and the anecdotal evidence that has been put forward is the notion of *superability*. Superability has been described as a 'weak' general motor ability, which underlies the learning and performance of *all* motor skills. It is the motor equivalent of general intelligence. The amount of superability that each person possesses will vary, just as people's Intelligence Quotient, the measure of general intelligence, does. Individuals with comparatively high levels of superability will be well disposed to learning many skills. However, each person also possesses many specific abilities. The person with low levels of superability but with a strong specific ability, may be good at some skills but weak at others.

The ability–skill interaction

In order to understand the ability–skill interaction, we can return to my breakdown of the skill of catching a ball. This time I will attempt to break it down in more detail, using actual abilities. The catcher must use coincidence-anticipation to determine the line, length and speed of flight. They must utilize hand–eye co-ordination to get their hands into position to catch the ball. If the ball is coming quickly they will need fast dynamic visual reaction time. In order to close their fingers around the ball they will require fast tactile reaction time.

By breaking down a fairly basic skill, as we have just done, it is possible to see that many abilities can affect performance. In more complex skills even more factors will be involved. As well as the large number of abilities that are involved in performing a skill, we must take into account the nature of the inter-relationship between these abilities. In Figure 1.2, I have used a method of diagrammatically describing the relevant importance of different abilities on the performance of a skill. I have taken the skill of dribbling in soccer as my example. In Figure 1.2(a), I show the relative importance of specific abilities for one player and in Figure 1.2(b) their relative importance for another player. These players are real people, both of whom I coached over several years. As can be seen from the two diagrams, the comparative importance of each ability differs yet both were equally good dribblers. However, the strength of each of their abilities differed and therefore, in order to be successful, they needed to dribble in different ways. There are many examples of this in top class sport. Both Goran Ivanisevic and André Agassi are good servers in tennis, but serve in

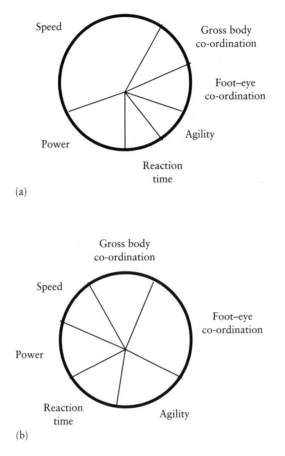

Figure 1.2 Skill–ability interaction: (a) shows the relative contribution of different abilities to skilful performance of dribbling by a professional soccer player; (b) demonstrates how the relative importance of each of these abilities differs in its contribution to the performance of another professional player

very different styles. I am sure that you can think of many examples from your own sports.

In order to further examine the ability–skill interaction, we need to be aware that the demands of a task are not necessarily constant. At the level of tennis played by Ivanisevic and Agassi, the serve needs to be fast and accurate or accurate and spinning. At lower levels of tennis simply being accurate may well suffice. At the beginner's level, it is not necessary to possess Ivanisevic's power or Agassi's guile. As the person moves up the levels of playing, the task changes and different abilities become more important. This is called the *changing task model*.

As well as the task changing as individuals step up from one level to another, the people themselves change. These changes may be developmental or due to practice. Examples of the individual changing would be factors like an increase in height or a change in morphology. The *changing person* factor is most noticeable as children go through puberty, but can also occur for other reasons, e.g., injuries can cause changes in the range of movement around a joint. This may mean that the individual has to alter the way he/she performs the skill.

The changing task and changing person factors make the use of testing abilities to predict future performance somewhat unreliable. This is exacerbated by the fact that different individuals use different abilities to produce the same end product. At the height of the Cold War both the Americans and the Soviet Bloc countries tried to use measurement of abilities to identify future stars, but with little success. Nevertheless, it is still used in some countries.

As more research has been undertaken into comparing elite and sub-elite performers we find that the differences in performance are sport specific rather than in specific abilities. A good example of this is research carried out by Janet Starkes comparing the Canadian Women's field hockey team with University and novice hockey players (Starkes, 1987). Starkes found that the internationals were only better than the other groups in hockey specific tests.

Summary

It is generally agreed that the performance of a skill is affected by what the individual brings to the task (abilities) and the demands of the task (nature of the skill). Moreover, it is accepted that abilities will change with time. Similarly, the nature of the skill will change when it is placed in a new context, e.g., playing against better opposition or using better equipment. It is also accepted that individuals will perform the same skill in different ways, depending on their own specific abilities. As a result, it is very difficult to use the measurement of abilities to predict performance.

Theories of performance

In this section, I will present a very brief overview of the theories of performance and learning that led to the development of Information Processing Theory and the ecological psychology theories. The early theories were based on animal studies and strongly featured the relationship between the stimulus and the response. According to the majority of these theories, when we want to satisfy some need or drive we search for a relevant stimulus and by trial and error discover what response will satisfy our need. These theories came from studies, such as Skinner's (1953), where animals were fed if they acted on a specific stimulus with a certain response. Gradually the relationship between the stimulus and the response was strengthened and the stimulus–response (S–R) bond was formed.

While these theories satisfied the behaviourists, those who tried to explain performance by what they observed, they were unsatisfactory as far as the cognitivists were concerned. The cognitivists were, as the name suggests, interested in the role of the brain in the learning and performance of skills. The first major group of cognitivists was the Gestältists. The Gestältists were concerned with the organization of perceptual behaviour into meaningful groups based on their inter-relationships. The individual uses this information to gain the necessary insight to aid problem solving. Problems are often solved by the person thinking through several possibilities before arriving at the correct answer.

Information Processing Theory

Although Gestält theories emphasized the role of cognition in performance, not all cognitivists were satisfied by the Gestältists' explanation of behaviour. It was too vague for many. This lack of satisfaction led to the development of *Information Processing Theory*. This theory was developed at the same time as computers and owes much to the theory of computing technology. The original attempt was as vague, if not more so, than the Gestältists. It is called the 'Black Box' model (see Figure 1.3). As can be seen from Figure 1.3, it explains very

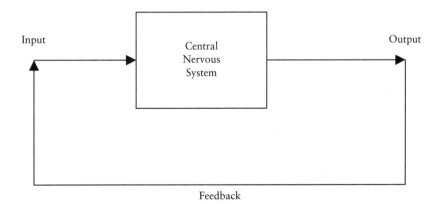

Figure 1.3   The 'Black Box' model of information processing

little about how we process information. In fact, it could be argued that it was a behaviourist theory because it concentrated on what happened rather than how it occurred. Information Processing Theory proper tried to remedy this.

Although there are many Information Processing models, they are basically the same. The model that can be seen in Figure 1.4 is a simplification of Welford's (1968) model. I will give a brief explanation of the model, then an outline of the criticisms made of it. It is up to the reader to evaluate the model and the criticisms as he/she reads the rest of this book. In deciding on the chapters of this book, I have followed Welford's divisions of information processing. This is for ease of organization and should not be taken to infer a preference for Information Processing Theory over ecological psychology theories. I have tried throughout the book to present both sides of the picture and, as I stated in the Prologue, it is up to the readers to make up their own minds as to which theory they prefer, if any.

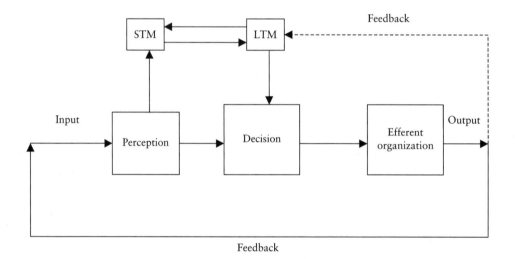

Figure 1.4 Model of information processing (adapted from Welford, 1968); reproduced by permission of Thomson Publishing Services from Welford, A.T. 1968 *Fundamentals of Skill*, Methuen, London, UK

The *input*, to which the Information Processing theorists refer, is all of the information present in the environment. It is sometimes referred to as the *display*. The display contains a vast amount of information, some relevant to the task and some irrelevant. Relevant information is often referred to as *relevant cues*, while irrelevant pieces of information are called *irrelevant cues*.

This information from the display is relayed to what we call the *Central Nervous System (CNS)*. The CNS is the brain, down to the second lumbar vertebrae. According to the Information Processing theorists, its role in performance is explained by the boxes or divisions shown in the model.

According to Information Processing Theory, the first role of the CNS is to interpret the incoming information. If we have normal senses we will all actually see, feel or hear the same things. However, the way in which we interpret them will differ. You only have to hear two people's accounts of the same incident to verify this. How we interpret the incoming information is the role of *perception*. Perhaps the major role of perception is to focus attention to task relevant cues at the expense of irrelevant ones. This is known as *selective attention*. The Information Processing theorists place great importance on the role of *memory* to aid perception and particularly selective attention.

Perception, according to the Information Processing theorists, is what we call *indirect*, i.e., it is dependent on our interpretation of the incoming information. This interpretation is based on a comparison between what we hold in *Short-term Memory (STM)* with what we hold in *Long-term Memory (LTM)*. As you can see from Figure 1.4, there are arrows going from STM to LTM and, also, arrows going the other way. The arrows going from STM to LTM represent the passing of information that we see, hear or feel in the environment from STM to LTM, where it can be stored for future use. The arrows from LTM to STM are concerned with performance rather than learning. The amount of information entering the CNS is vast, therefore we must have some way of selecting the cues to which we will attend. It is thought that this is particularly important, as we are limited in the amount of information with which we can deal at any one moment in time. I am sure that, at this moment in time, some of you are saying 'you're telling me'! The ability to determine which cues are relevant takes place in the STM. The arrows from the LTM to the STM show how this happens. When people find themselves in a familiar situation, they transfer past experience about such situations from the LTM to the STM. Thus, the STM is forewarned of what is relevant and what is irrelevant, allowing the person to selectively attend to the relevant cues.

This comparison of information, held in the STM and LTM, not only allows the individual to make sense of the incoming information – perception – it also allows the person to decide what action to take in any given situation – *Decision Making*. These processes together are often referred to as *working memory*. Once a decision has been taken of what action to make, the CNS has to organize the movement (*Efferent Organization*). The information, concerning movement organization, is sent from the CNS to the *Peripheral Nervous System (PNS)*, so that the movement can take place. Once we start to move, we begin to process *feedback*. Feedback can be information about the nature of our movements. In Figure 1.4, this is depicted by the bottom feedback arrow. In slow movements, we can use this information to alter or refine our actions as they are being carried out. The top feedback arrow represents information about the success or failure of our actions, and is fed back to memory. This information is stored in LTM and is responsible for learning.

Throughout this book, we will examine the criticisms of Information Processing Theory. At this stage, it will suffice to outline the major criticisms. The fact that this process is so dependent on memory, in particular the interaction between STM and LTM, means that it must be time consuming. There are many instances in real life which occur much faster than those that can be accounted for by Information Processing Theory. Sport provides many fine examples of this. Normal reaction time, as found in laboratory studies, ranges between 170 and 200 milliseconds (ms). This is simple reaction time, when there is only one stimulus and one response. If we increase the numbers of possible stimuli and responses, reaction time increases dramatically. In fast ball games, the player often has very little time in which to respond to a stimulus. There are many examples of this and I will give two here. A cricket batter, facing a bowler bowling at 140 km/h (80 mph), has approximately 500 ms in which to decide what shot to play *and* actually play the shot. Similarly a soccer goalkeeper, facing a penalty kick hit at 100 km/h (55 mph), has only 440 ms in which to save the ball. If Information Processing Theory were correct, it would be impossible for a goalkeeper to save a penalty or a batter to hit the ball. The Information Processing theorists argue that such actions can only take place if the batter or goalkeeper uses *anticipation*. There is some support for this claim (see Chapter 5); nevertheless it does leave some questions unanswered.

Another major criticism that has been made of Information Processing Theory is that, if perception and decision were dependent on the STM–LTM interaction, individuals would only be capable of producing responses for which they have some form of past experience. Thus, the theory cannot account for novel actions. The Information Processing theorists counter this argument by stating that all the individual needs is experience of a similar, not necessarily the same, situation. The person can then compare the similarities and dissimilarities of the present situation, held in STM, with the past experience, stored in LTM, before deciding how to act. Schmidt's (1975) Schema Theory (see Chapter 8) attempts to explain this by stating that we do not hold actual past experiences in memory but rather basic rules or schemas (sometimes called schemata) concerning our actions.

The third major criticism of Information Processing Theory is concerned with Efferent Organization. The critics argue that, if the CNS were responsible for the organization of all actions that we take, we would need a much larger brain than we have. The Information Processing theorists claim that, once we have learned a movement, we store what they call a *motor program* (the efferent organization for the movement) and this motor program can trigger movement with a minimum of effort and organization. Critics counteract this claim by stating that, even if motor programs require little in the nature of attention and are automatic, we are able to carry out so many skills that we would still need a massive brain to store all the motor programs. As a result of this criticism, the Information Processing theorists modified their theory to claim that we do not store each separate motor program but that we store a *generalized motor program* and are able to modify each general program for each specific situation. Recently, many Information Processing theorists have accepted that the CNS may only organize the major aspects of the movement and the PNS may be responsible for refining it, to control for the specifics of the situation. We will cover this, and the other major criticisms of Information Processing Theory, in the relevant chapters later in this book.

Ecological psychology theories

The biggest critics of Information Processing Theory have been the ecological psychologists. While Information Processing Theory had its conception in cognitive theories of psychology, the ecological psychologists were concerned with what could be observed rather than what was inferred. As such they were more based in the behaviourist school. The founding fathers of ecological psychology were the Russian Nikolaï Bernstein and the American J. J. Gibson. Gibson (1979) was concerned with how well we could account for performance based on scientific laws and humans' interaction with nature. His ideas developed into Action Systems Theory. At the same time that Gibson was developing his beliefs, Bernstein was independently developing his. Bernstein's (1967) ideas were wider in scope than Gibson's but followed the same principle of trying to explain action with as little reference as possible to the role of the CNS. Bernstein and Gibson did not deny that the CNS has a role to play in performance but they claimed that, as we can only speculate what that role is, reference to it is non-scientific. We should use scientific principles to explain movement. As far as Bernstein was concerned, these scientific principles could come from physics, Darwinian evolution theory, biology or any other branch of science.

Although there are several ecological psychology theories, the two that have received the greatest amount of attention are *Action Systems Theory* and *Dynamical Systems Theory*. These theories complement one another and, therefore, in recent years they have tended to be treated as one or, at least, both are used to explain behaviour by ecological psychologists. Therefore, in this text we will use the term ecological psychology when discussing points that are covered by both theories. If an argument is put forward by only one of the theories we will use the name of that specific theory.

Ecological psychology places great emphasis on the interaction between humans and the environment. The environment dictates what we are allowed to do at any given time in any specific situation. Gibson called these opportunities for action and gave them the name *'affordances'*. Moreover, no two situations are exactly the same, therefore affordances may be similar but never identical. While affordances are present at all times, they will not be acted upon if the individual is unaware of their existence. The person must *actively search* the environment or display for the presence of affordances. A good, though still painful for me, example of this came about when I was coaching a professional soccer team in an important game. The centre-forward had the ball in the centre of the field about 40 m from goal. The right-side midfield player was marked, but the left-side midfield player had a free run to goal. Thus the situation provided an affordance to pass the ball to the left-hand side thus allowing the left-side midfielder to head for goal. The centre-forward, however, only looked to the right. He was aware that he could pass the ball to the right-side midfield player. This he did. Unfortunately, this player lost the ball when tackled. The centre-forward was not aware of the affordance to pass the ball to the unmarked left-side midfield player because he had not examined the left side of the display. We lost the game 1–0. I did not bother explaining to the centre-forward that affordances can only be perceived and acted upon if we actively search for them.

Had the centre-forward searched the display fully, he would have recognized the affordance to pass to the unmarked left-side midfield player and made the correct response. To the Information Processing theorists, this would be because he would have recalled similar situations from his LTM and known that this would bring success. The ecological psychologists dispute this. They agree that the centre-forward would have perceived the affordance and made the correct decision but because the information necessary to make the correct decision was present in the display directly. There was *no need for memory*. If the player understood the goals of soccer, to score, he would perceive the affordance. As long as he searched for it, that is. This is called *direct perception*.

Sport provides many examples of direct perception. As long as you know the aims or goals of the game, the environment provides the necessary opportunities for actions. If you had never played tennis before but saw that your opponent was at one side of the court, you would not need past experience to see the affordance of playing a shot to other side of the court. I am sure that you can provide similar examples from your own sports.

The above account, of direct perception of affordances, may give some readers the impression that the ecological psychologists, like the Information Processing theorists, believe that perception precedes action. They do not subscribe to such a division, which they see as being arbitrary. According to them, perception and action are linked. This is called *perception–action coupling*. In order to perceive the relevant affordances, the person must act upon the environment. He/she must actively search the environment, using afferent (sensory) and efferent (motor) nerves. Thus perception of the affordance is dependent on movement, as much as receiving sensory information. My centre-forward did not perceive the affordance because he did not move his head, so that he could see the left-hand side of the display. Similarly, once a person begins to act, it is both perception and action that control movement. In other words, as we move we use sensory information to help us control that movement. When running, you move your legs and arms but you also look to see where you are going. You are even aware of the feel of your movement.

This does not appear to be too different from the Information Processing Theory explanation of the use of feedback to control slow movements. Ecological psychologists do not like that explanation, as they see it as referring to a CNS function which we can not be sure happens. Moreover, they argue that as afferent and efferent nerves are inter-connected in the spinal cord, it may be at PNS level that movement is controlled rather than in the CNS. We discuss this argument in some detail in Chapter 7.

The ecological psychologists' explanation of the control of movement differs quite markedly from that of the Information Processing theorists. According to ecological psychologists, the role of the CNS is merely to decide what action to take. The CNS then provides a very broad set of commands. These commands are said to be *functionally specific*. They are as simple as 'catch the ball' or 'kick the ball'. It is the role of perception–action coupling to determine exactly how the command is carried out, i.e., the way in which we kick the ball, whether it is with the instep, inside or outside of the foot. The perception–action coupling found in any given situation is unique to that situation and will depend on what is required to achieve the chosen goal. Thus, there is no need for motor programs.

While the theory of motor programs states that the movement of, and interaction between, limbs is organized by the CNS, Dynamical Systems Theory states that the PNS organizes limb movements. This organization is not dependent on memory or detailed instructions from the CNS but is the result of the interaction between limbs that are obeying scientific laws. Thus, it is said that the organism is capable of *'self-organization'*. If you lean to your right, your left arm and leg will automatically move to make sure that you do not fall over. Similarly, if you bend your arm your biceps tense but your triceps relax. If they did not, you would not be able to bend your arm.

The organization of movement is determined by personal and environmental factors. How each person organizes their movements will differ because of their individual strengths and weaknesses. They will, in fact, perform the same skill differently. As we pointed out earlier in this chapter, Michael Johnson and Maurice Greene use different styles when running. This is because they are organismically different. Similarly, environmental factors, such as weather conditions, will result in the movement being organized in different ways. It requires a different movement to control a hockey ball on astroturf compared with on grass. Another example is having to run uphill or downhill for that matter. Both require different techniques from running on the flat.

In outlining ecological psychology theories, I have introduced some of the terminology used by the ecological psychologists. However, I have deliberately not mentioned many of them. They can be somewhat difficult to understand and are often misleading. Therefore, I will wait until later in the book to introduce more of them. Some I have not used at all in the text. In Appendix 2, I have provided a glossary of such terms.

Two major criticisms of ecological psychology theories have been postulated. The first is that the refusal to accept the role of memory in performance appears to be contradictory to common sense. It is obvious, from observation of individuals, that they develop their ability to carry out tasks through practice. If the organism were self-organizing, without recourse to memory or some form of internal representation, the person would be able to perform the task equally as well the first time as subsequent times. This we know is not the case. Very few ecological psychologists now hold the view that some form of internal representation does not take place. They are, however, reluctant to use the word memory, e.g., the development of the ability to perceive affordances is called 'attunement to affordances'.

The second major criticism of ecological psychology is its failure to account for cognitive processes, e.g., decision making. Although ecological psychologists claim that we become attuned to affordances through experience of similar situations, they do not account for how we decide which affordance is the most suitable in any given situation. Anyone involved in sport knows that players often choose an action that is less than optimal. The example that I gave earlier of the centre-forward not passing to the left-side midfield player was due to a failure to perceive the affordance. However, the same player often made incorrect choices even when he had searched the whole display. Ecological psychology makes no attempt to explain how this occurs.

Conclusion

While some psychologists vehemently support their own 'pet' theory, the majority accepts that neither theory can totally explain skilled performance. By and large, psychologists can be divided into three camps: those who believe that the best explanation of behaviour is likely to come from the refinement of Information Processing Theory; those who think it lies in the development of ecological psychology; and those who believe in a hybrid theory, taking the best from each school of thought. Many believe that Information Processing Theory provides the best explanation of decision making, while ecological psychology explains movement better. There is, however, less consensus concerning the different explanations of perception – the direct versus inferred debate.

The reason that neither theory has been unanimously accepted by psychologists may be due to the fact that *both* provide explanations of how we perform skills. So far psychologists have not been able to find skills that can only be explained by one theory and not the other.

Key points

Skill

- Skill may be objectively measured, based on the outcome regardless of the aesthetic merits of the performance.

- Skill may be measured qualitatively, based on what it looks like to the observer.

- Skills may be classified along a continuum from fine (involving few limbs) to gross (involving many limbs).

- Skill may be defined as discrete (having a definite beginning and end), serial (a number of discrete skills linked together) or continuous (having no definite beginning or end).

- Skills may be defined as being simple (containing little in the way of perception and decision making) or complex (drawing heavily on perception and decision making).

- Skills may be classified along a continuum from open (taking place in an ever-changing environment) to closed (taking place in an environment that rarely changes).

Ability

- Abilities are innate.

- Abilities can be improved by practice but only to a limited extent.

- The main theories of ability are:

  - general motor ability (determines the individual's prowess at all sports),

  - Henry's specificity hypothesis (abilities are unique and bear no relationship to one another),

  - Fleishman's factor analysis hypothesis (abilities can be grouped into clusters, which have low to moderate correlations with one another),

  - superability (a weak general motor ability underpinning the individual's prowess at sport, but this is also affected by specific abilities).

Ability–skill interaction

- Abilities underpin the performance of skills.

- Different people perform the same skill in different ways because they possess different abilities.

- The relative importance of different abilities change over time:

  - changing task model (the nature of the skill changes as we move from beginner to elite performer),

  - changing person model (the way in which we perform a skill changes due to changes in our abilities).

Information Processing Theory

- The Information Processing Theory model (see Figure 1.4) consists of:

  - perception (what we make of the information around us),

  - decision making (what action we decide to take),

  - memory (STM and LTM),

  - efferent organization (the organization of the movements that we wish to make),

  - proprioceptive feedback (aids the control of slow movements),

  - feedback for learning.

- Perception is indirect or inferred and is dependent on memory.

- Decision making is dependent on the comparison of the present situation, held in STM, with similar past experiences stored in LTM.

- Perception–memory–decision making form working memory.

- Well-learned skills are stored as motor programs.

- The PNS merely relays information to and from the CNS:

  - information to the CNS is relayed via sensory or afferent nerves,

  - information from the CNS is relayed by motor or efferent nerves,

  - sensory nerves are responsible for perception,

  - motor nerves are responsible for action.

- The major criticisms of the theory are:

  - the process described would be very time consuming and would take longer than the time taken to perform many skills,

- ○ it does not account for the performance of novel skills,

- ○ our brains are not large enough to store all the motor programs we would need.

Ecological psychology theories

- The major ecological psychology theories are Action Systems Theory and Dynamical Systems Theory.

- The CNS is responsible for deciding our goal (what we wish to do) in any given situation:

  - ○ this decision is very general and is said to be functionally specific, e.g., catch the ball, kick the ball.

- We actively search the environment for affordances (opportunities to achieve our goal).

- Perception is direct; it does not require memory, all of the information necessary is present in the environment.

- Perception and action are coupled (both work together to help us perceive and act upon the affordances):

  - ○ sensory and motor nerves are responsible for perception,

  - ○ sensory and motor nerves are responsible for action.

- Movement is controlled by the PNS:

  - ○ it is self-organizing (muscles, joints and nerves interact with one another to create the movement).

Test your knowledge

(Answers in Appendix 3.)

Part one

Choose which of the phrases, (a), (b), (c) or (d), is the most accurate. There is only *one* correct answer for each problem.

1. An example of a serial skill is:

    (a) putting the shot,

    (b) the triple jump,

    (c) the front crawl,

    (d) kicking a soccer ball.

2. The basketball set shot is an example of a:

    (a) discrete skill,

    (b) serial skill,

    (c) continuous skill,

    (d) perceptual skill.

3. According to Henry, reaction time is a:

    (a) general ability,

    (b) specific ability,

    (c) continuous skill,

    (d) technique.

4. Abilities:

    (a) cannot be improved by practice,

    (b) are hereditary,

    (c) are not affected by age,

    (d) can be improved dramatically by practice.

5. Superability is:

(a) an ability that is better than the person's general ability level,

(b) an ability that allows the person to become a top-class athlete,

(c) a strong general motor ability,

(d) a weak general motor ability.

6. As children develop physically, the way in which they perform a skill may change because:

(a) their abilities alter,

(b) the task alters,

(c) they learn faster,

(d) they become more motivated.

7. According to Information Processing Theory, perception is dependent on:

(a) short-term memory only,

(b) long-term memory only,

(c) both short- and long-term memory,

(d) attunement to affordances.

8. According to Information Processing Theory, efferent nerves:

(a) are responsible for initiating movement,

(b) are set in motion by the PNS,

(c) provide proprioceptive feedback,

(d) are also called sensory nerves.

9. Which of the following is not accounted for by Information Processing Theory?

(a) performing skills automatically,

(b) the production of novel responses,

(c) performing more than one skill at a time,

(d) performing skills without recourse to feedback.

10. According to ecological psychology, movement is:

(a) organized by efferent organization in the CNS,

(b) organized by the muscles and joints,

(c) dependent on motor memory,

(d) dependent on working memory.

11. According to ecological psychology, perception is not possible without:

(a) action,

(b) experience,

(c) knowledge,

(d) working memory.

12. Which of the following is not well explained by ecological psychology theories?

(a) how we can perform very fast movements,

(b) how we can perform skills that require a great deal of co-ordination,

(c) how we can perform different variations of the same skill,

(d) how we make decisions.

Part two

Which of the following statements are true (T) and which are false (F)?

1.	Skill must be learned explicitly.	T	F
2.	A skill does not have to be aesthetically pleasing.	T	F
3.	The outcome of a skill must be measured quantitatively.	T	F
4.	Passing a ball, in a basketball game, is a complex skill.	T	F
5.	Passing a ball, in a basketball game, is a discrete skill.	T	F

6. A person can have a relatively weak superability but still be good at a particular sport.   T   F

7. The relative importance of different abilities, when performing a skill, can change as we move from one level of competition to another.   T   F

8. Having good technique does not necessarily mean that we are skilful.   T   F

9. By measuring the ability levels of children, we can easily predict who will be good at different sports when they become adults.   T   F

10. Working memory consists of perception, short-term memory, decision making and recall from long-term memory.   T   F

11. According to Information Processing Theory, efferent organization is responsible for every part of a movement.   T   F

12. The efferent nerves are also known as the motor nerves.   T   F

13. Information Processing Theory is good at explaining how we can perform movements of less than one reaction time.   T   F

14. According to Information Processing Theory, motor programs are the result of lots of practice.   T   F

15. According to ecological psychology theories, instructions from the CNS, concerning what action to take, are detailed.   T   F

16. According to ecological psychology theories, perception is passive.   T   F

17. Action Systems theorists say that perception is direct because it does not require memory.   T   F

18. According to Dynamical Systems Theory, perception precedes action.   T   F

19. According to Dynamical Systems Theory, the PNS plays little role in the organization of movement.   T   F

20. According to Action Systems Theory, movement is self-organized.   T   F

Additional reading

Billing J (1980) Overview of task complexity. *Motor Skills: Theory into Practice* 4: 18–23

Fairweather M (1999) Skill learning principles: implications for coaching practice. In: *The coaching process*, Cross N and Lyle J (Eds) Butterworth Heinemann, Oxford, UK, pp. 113–129

Mechling HH (1999) Co-ordinative abilities. In: *Psychology for physical educators*, Vanden Auweele Y *et al.* (Eds) Human Kinetics, Champaign, Illinois, USA, pp. 159–186

Sugden D (2002) Moving forward to dynamic choices: David Sugden, University of Leeds, PEAUK Fellow Lecture, 4 December 2001. *Brit J Teaching Phys Educ* 33: 6–8; 25

2 Perception

Acquisition and Performance of Sports Skills   T. McMorris
© 2004 John Wiley & Sons, Ltd   ISBNs: 0-470-84994-0 (HB); 0-470-84995-9 (PB)

Introduction

In this chapter we examine, from an Information Processing perspective, the role of perception in working memory, i.e., how perception aids decision making. From an ecological psychology standpoint, we are looking at how perception and action combine to recognize the existence of affordances in the environment. The role of perception in the control of movement is covered in Chapter 7.

Information Processing Theory and perception

Although Information Processing theorists argue that *sensation* and *perception* are different, the two concepts tend to be treated as one. The senses, which are the most important in the perception of information present in the environment, are visual and auditory receptors. Vision is generally considered to be the most important of the senses. Light waves are detected by the retina and transduced to nerve impulses, which are transmitted to the CNS, in particular to the sensory cortex. The central portion of the eye, the *fovea*, is rich in nerve receptors, which allow it to extract detail from an object. The range of *foveal* or *central vision* depends on how the eye is focused. This is controlled by the *ciliary muscle*. The range is generally regarded as being between 2° and 5°. The vision outside of this range is referred to as *peripheral vision*. The receptors, here, are less dense and images are less distinct than those found in foveal vision.

Although foveal and peripheral vision are commonly used terms, Trevarthen (1968) used the terms *focal* and *ambient vision*. Focal vision is identical to foveal vision, but ambient vision differs a little from peripheral vision. According to Trevarthen, ambient vision includes visual information from both the fovea and periphery. The information coming from foveal vision, however, is not what the individual is focusing on but the other light rays which are being detected. As such, these images will be less distinct than those focused on by the fovea (those in focal vision) and will be similar in distinctiveness to the images from the periphery. Thus, it is argued that there are two visual processes providing information about our environment. *Audition* can also supply useful information to the performer, e.g., good table tennis players can pick up a great deal of information, about how much spin an opponent has placed on the ball, by the sound of bat–ball contact.

According to Information Processing Theory, the senses merely transmit information about the environment to the CNS. The information provided by the senses to the CNS is, in itself, meaningless. It is the CNS that interprets the information and makes sense of it. Perception, therefore, is said to be *indirect* or *inferred*. By this, we mean that the senses relay meaningless nerve impulses to the CNS, which *organizes* and *interprets* the information. The ability to organize and interpret the information is based on past experience held in LTM. This information is compared to the present situation, which is stored in the STM. The individual can only utilize the sensory information after carrying out this comparison. Only then, can they organize and interpret the information. An experienced table tennis player can determine the amount of spin placed on a ball from hearing the sound made at bat–ball contact. To an inexperienced person this information is meaningless.

The interpretation of the perceptual information regarding the amount of spin placed on the ball by the table tennis player would not be determined solely by sound. The player would also take into account what he/she saw – the point of bat–ball contact, the movement of the bat before and after contact, the position of forearms compared to upper arms and possibly even facial expressions. Thus, perception depends on the *integration* of sensory information.

Based on the above, we can define perception, according to Information Processing Theory, as being *the organization, interpretation and integration of sensory information*. Kerr (1982) provides a similar definition but includes the word 'conscious'. Although Information Processing theorists would argue that most of the time perception is a conscious process, recent research on learning and anticipation has shown that it can take place at a sub-conscious level.

Signal Detection Theory

As Information Processing Theory claims that perception is inferred, a number of theories have been developed to explain different aspects of the cognitive processes taking place. One of the first theories was Swets' (1964; Swets and Green, 1964) *Signal Detection Theory*. Swets realized that people live in an environment which is full of sensory information. He reckoned that an individual receives over 100 000 signals/s. These may be signals from the environment and/or from within the person themselves. Sport provides many examples of this and the problems it can cause. Think of a tennis player about to serve in a game on the Centre Court at Wimbledon. What kinds of signals do you think the player will be receiving visually and auditorally? What kinds of internal signals might the player be receiving, e.g., will I win, will I play well? The problem facing Swets was how to explain how anyone can recognize relevant information against this background of signals, which he termed *'noise'*.

According to Signal Detection Theory, the probability of detecting any given stimulus or signal depends on the *intensity of the signal compared with the intensity of the background noise*. Swets claimed that noise is present constantly but varies in intensity from time to time. He said that the average amount of noise could be described by a normal bell curve, where the mean level of noise is represented by the central portion of the curve. Any incoming signal, the stimulus to be detected, increases the amount of neural activity. This he represented by two bell curves, one depicting noise only the other depicting the noise *plus* the signal (see Figure 2.1).

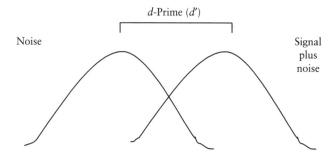

Figure 2.1 Graphic description of Signal Detection Theory (adapted from Swets and Green, 1964)

The likelihood of detecting the signal would depend on the interaction between two variables, *d*-prime (*d'*) and the criterion (*C*). *d'* represents the individual's *sensitivity* to that particular signal. This sensitivity may be sensory, e.g., visual acuity, auditory acuity. It may also depend on experience, e.g., familiar signals are thought to be more readily detected than unfamiliar stimuli. Swets depicted the differences in the sensitivity of *d'* by the distance between the peaks of the noise only and noise plus signal bell curves (see Figure 2.1).

Signal Detection Theory, however, states that the probability of detection is also affected by *C*. *C* represents the affect of a person's *bias* on detection. Figure 2.2 diagrammatically demonstrates this effect. The criterion *C* is thought to be affected by arousal level, which in turn affects the probability of the detection of a signal. When *C* is depicted too far to the right, and the signal is missed (*omission*), this is because arousal is low. If, however, *C* is depicted as being too far to the left, arousal is high and detection is considered to be a high priority, of too much importance in fact. As a result the individual may perceive a signal

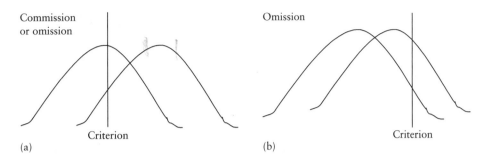

Figure 2.2 Graphic description of the effect of changes in the criterion (C) on signal detection (adapted from Swets, 1964)

when one does not exist (*commission*). They may, also, be unable to detect the signal from the background because the noise is too great, as a result of an increase caused by their internal worries and fears.

Swets' use of bell curves may cause some of you problems in understanding Signal Detection Theory. The basic psychology underpinning the theory is, in fact, quite simple. The signal/background interaction is seen many times in sport. Sightscreens are used in cricket to help the batter perceive the ball against the background. Table tennis players are not allowed to wear white, as it will make it difficult for their opponent to detect the white ball against the colour of their clothes. This aspect of signal detection is often overlooked in sport. In cricket a red ball is still used in daytime games, yet it is very difficult for the fielders to detect against the background of spectators. It is difficult for the spectators to see it at all. This was demonstrated to me very graphically a number of years ago. I watched a cricket Test Match at Edgbaston and had great difficulty in perceiving the ball when the fast bowlers were in action. A few days later, I attended a Toronto Blue Jays baseball game in the Sky Dome. Roger Clements, the fastest pitcher in the World at that time, was pitching for Toronto. I was concerned that I would not be able to see the ball. I need not have worried. Despite the fact that he was pitching faster than the bowlers at Edgbaston, I could see the ball against the background of the spectators because it was white.

While colour of the ball against the background is a good example of the signal/background interaction, it can also be an example of d'. If a person is colour blind this will affect their sensitivity to certain signal/background contrasts. Similarly poor eyesight or hearing can affect this sensitivity. Research, however, has shown that there are differences in sensitivity even between individual's who possess good vision or audition. It would appear that familiarity with the signal is the key factor. On the first occasion that I played cricket against a good leg spin bowler, I was totally unable to detect which ball was a leg spinner and which a top spinner. My team-mates, who were more experienced than me, had no such difficulty.

Pattern recognition

The example, given above, concerning the ability of a cricket batter to detect the type of ball that is being bowled, leads us to consider another aspect of signal detection. In situations where the performer has limited time in which to make a response such as batting in baseball, it is of little use to the batter if he/she can only detect the signal *after* the ball has been pitched. In these situations, the batter needs to be able to detect what kind of ball is being delivered *before* the ball has left the pitcher's hand. As we will see in Chapter 5, there is plenty of evidence to show that it is possible for expert performers to perceive a signal from only partial information. This is called *pattern recognition*. This pattern recognition allows the batter to anticipate the line of flight and so hit even a fast ball.

   In order to utilize pattern recognition, the performer must be able to perceive some regularity in the patterns of stimuli that he/she is seeing. The perception of the pattern allows the player to determine what kind of ball has been pitched before the entire signal has been seen. Figure 2.3 shows a tennis player playing

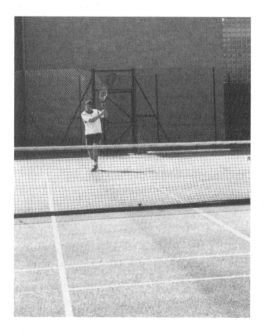

Figure 2.3   What kind of shot is the player playing – down the line or cross-court?

a forehand shot. Can you tell whether it is a cross-court or down the line shot from the position of his body?

A slightly different aspect of pattern recognition is the phenomenon known as *closure*. A good example of closure occurs when we see an object moving towards us, but then lose sight of it for a brief period of time, due to some obstruction to our view. We are able to judge when and where it will reappear by mentally 'filling in the gap' in our visual tracking. Cricket wicket-keepers do this when the ball passes down the leg side of the batter and he/she momentarily blocks their view. This ability to 'fill in' the gap is closure. The 'filling in' of the line of flight and the ability to perceive familiar patterns is, according to Information Processing Theory, the result of experience. It is a CNS function and takes place in working memory.

Selective attention

I think that most readers will readily understand why it is important to be able to recognize patterns so that we can anticipate where a ball is going. In fast ball games, for example, it is obvious just from observation and, even more so, from participation that we cannot wait to see the entire signal before deciding what response to make. The importance of limiting the number of signals or stimuli to which we attend – *selective attention* – may be less obvious. As Signal Detection Theory states, we are constantly being bombarded by information. However, we do not and cannot process all the stimuli we are receiving at any one moment in time. How limited we are in being able to deal with more than one signal at a time is a matter of some debate. In fact, the first theory put forward with regard to this problem claimed that we can deal only with *one* piece of information at a time (Welford, 1968).

Welford stated that the process from detection of the stimulus to the beginning of producing a response was a *single-channel* operation. According to Welford, the only way that we are able to do more than one thing at a time is to switch attention between different pieces of information. Although Welford later modified his theory to state that automatic actions, e.g., walking and running, could take place at the same time as the processing of other information, he pointed to reaction-time research to provide support for his theory.

The types of research that Welford used to support his theory were research into the psychological refractory period (see Chapter 4) and dual-task research. Dual-task research concerns the doing of two things at the same time. Early research showed that when people were measured on their performance on two tasks, their performance was significantly better when each task was performed separately, compared with when they tried to do both tasks at the same time. Welford claimed that this supported his theory.

You can carry out your own dual-task experiment very simply. Make two 6 cm squares and place them 10 cm apart. See how many times you can touch each square in 30 s, using your preferred hand. Get someone to write down a series of lists of two digit numbers (10 numbers per series). You will need about 10 lists. Give yourself 30 s to add up as many series as possible. Check how accurate you were and how many series you completed. Try to do both tasks at the same time. Compare your scores for each task, when done separately and when carried out simultaneously. Another test is to throw a tennis ball, using your preferred hand, at a target (a 50 cm square) 6 m away from you. See how many accurate throws you can make in 1 min. This is task one. For task two, bounce a basketball, with your non-dominant hand, into a 1 m square as many times as you can in 1 min. Try to do both tasks at the same time.

For most of you, scores when doing one task will be better than when doing both together. However, this will not necessarily be the case. Welford would expect that those of you who are regular basketball players would be able to do that task with little conscious effort, therefore performance on the two tasks would not be significantly affected. Even where this is not the case, some of you will not have been negatively affected by doing two tasks at once.

Several researchers have found that dual-task performance has not necessarily resulted in interference in performance. This led theorists to question single-channel theory. Research that has found that doing two tasks at the same time does not result in deterioration in performance has generally utilized two tasks that are very dissimilar. It is said that such tasks *require different pathways*. So in our experiment, it may be that the maths task and the hand-tapping task did not significantly affect one another. This is because they use different CNS and PNS pathways. One would expect the two ball tasks to be negatively affected, as there is some use of the same pathways. Findings such as these led to the development of *multi-channel theory*. According to multi-channel theory, we have several channels, each dealing with different types of task. In addition, the multi-channel theorists claimed that we have a *superordinate channel*. This superordinate channel is able to carry out cognitive tasks, such as decision making, while the other channels take care of motor tasks.

Like single-channel theory, multi-channel theories are what we call *fixed capacity* theories. By this we mean that each channel has a capacity that does not alter with the situation. Deutsch and Deutsch (1963) claimed that we could do more than one thing without deterioration in performance, as long as the demands on attention do not exceed the limitations of the channel. They pointed, in particular, to performing two acts when one of them is automatic.

Alternatives to fixed capacity theories are *flexible capacity* theories. The best known flexible capacity theory is Kahneman's (1973) *allocatable resources theory*. The explanation of how we do more than one thing at a time is very similar to that used by Deutsch and Deutsch. However, according to Kahneman the capacity, or *pool of resources*, is not fixed. Kahneman believes that the capacity changes as arousal changes. So an increase in arousal results in an increase in the number of resources available. The key factor is how the individual allocates these resources. The allocation of the resources is said to be the role of what Kahneman terms *cognitive effort*. This is discussed in more detail in Chapter 10.

Regardless of which theory we support, it is certain that we have a limited capacity, whether fixed or flexible, and that doing more than one thing at a time causes problems. Moreover, *we are not able to attend to all the stimuli in the environment*. Therefore, we must somehow blot out attention to irrelevant stimuli. The first person to attempt to explain how this occurs was Donald Broadbent (1958). Broadbent said that *all* information enters the STM, but that we only attend to selected stimuli. In other words, only selected information is compared to information stored in LTM. The stimuli are said to pass through a *selective filter*, which allows only chosen information to be accessible to the LTM (Figure 2.4).

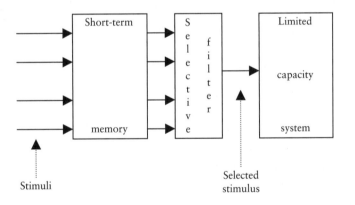

Figure 2.4 Broadbent's filter model of selective attention (adapted from Broadbent, 1958)

Broadbent's theory is an 'all or nothing' theory, i.e., if a stimulus is not selected, it will not pass through the filter and so will not be attended to. Ann Treisman (1964) pointed out that this is not always the case. She argued that, although we may consciously choose a stimulus or set of stimuli to which to attend, we do not lose awareness of all the other information. Like Broadbent, Treisman claimed that all information enters the selective filter and the selected information is processed by working memory. However, she states that the non-selected information is what she terms *'attenuated'*. If the attenuated stimuli are unfamiliar they will be discarded, as suggested by Broadbent. However, if the attenuated information is familiar, it will still be processed. Supporters of Treisman point to Cherry's cocktail party effect to support this claim. Cherry's (1953) experiments on attention showed that familiar stimuli would be attended to sub-consciously. He claimed that this was exemplified by what happens if we are in a crowded room and engaged in conversation with friends, such as at a cocktail party. We are unaware of what is being said in other conversations unless someone happens to mention our name. We are not consciously listening for our name but, because it is a familiar stimulus, we still hear it.

Norman (1969) provided a similar model to that of Treisman except that he argued that the key factor in attention was not familiarity but *pertinence*. Norman argued that it is how important the stimulus is to the task at hand that will determine whether or not we attend to it (Figure 2.5). An example of this would be a hockey player in possession of the ball. The player may be looking ahead of him/herself for someone to pass the ball to, when they suddenly become aware of a defender approaching them from the side. This latter information is processed because of its pertinence. To ignore it would result in losing the ball.

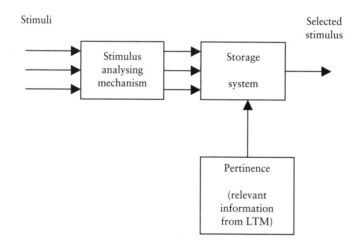

Figure 2.5   Norman's model of selective attention (adapted from Norman, 1969)

While the above models try to provide an explanation of how we block out irrelevant information and point to the fact that we attempt to attend to relevant information, they do not explain how we determine what is relevant and what is not. Information Processing theorists claim that the decision is due to past experience. As we experience different situations we store, in LTM, the results of our actions and which information was useful to us. When we find ourselves in similar situations, at a later date, we recall that information and search the environment for the information, or cues, that we perceive as being relevant. Cues that are not deemed to be relevant are blocked by the selective filter.

Visual search

As we stated in the last section, we search the environment for cues that we believe are relevant to the task in hand. Research by Fran Allard and colleagues (Allard and Starkes, 1980; Allard, Graham and Paarsalu, 1980) showed that experts and novices carried out their searches in different ways. Using eye mark recorders, they examined the search patterns of experienced and inexperienced basketball and volleyball players. They found that the experts, in the two games, followed very similar patterns of search, even though the displays in the two games differ a great deal. The experts looked firstly at spaces behind defenders, then at the positions of the defenders and lastly at the positions of their team-mates. The novices, also, followed similar patterns to one another but these patterns were very different to those used by the experts. In fact, they were the other way round. According to Allard, this was due to past experience showing the experts which information was the most important.

Although the key factor in determining the effectiveness of visual search is the decision concerning which stimuli to attend to, there are also genetic limit-ations, similar to the abilities examined in Chapter 1. These genetic factors affect visual search, or rather its efficiency. In the following paragraphs we will look very briefly at these factors. More detail can be found in any basic human biology text covering vision.

One of the major factors affecting visual search in sport is the *span of apprehension*. This refers to the amount of information the individual can perceive in one glance. It would appear that having a large span of apprehen-sion is advantageous. This, however, will only be the case if the person has good selective attention. A large span of apprehension helps us not to miss vital cues but it also means that there will be more irrelevant information in the display than if the span were small.

The span of apprehension will be affected by the range of peripheral vision. We tend to think of peripheral vision as referring to what we can perceive from the 'corners' of the eyes, i.e., *horizontal* peripheral vision. It should be remembered that peripheral vision also has a *vertical* component. A large range of horizontal peripheral vision allows us to be aware of what is happening to our right and left, something very important in most sports. A large range of vertical peripheral vision is particularly useful in sports like soccer and hockey where, when in possession of the ball, the performer needs to be aware of the position of the ball and the position of opponents and team-mates.

While the comments made above may seem to be obvious, research comparing the range of peripheral vision of sports people and non-sports people tends to show no significant differences. The majority of this research, however, has examined *static* peripheral vision. In general, research has shown that static *visual acuity* is not a key factor in sports performance. However, there does appear to be an advantage in possessing good *dynamic* visual acuity. It has been shown that individuals differ in their ability to track moving objects, particularly when the object is moving at speed. When we track slow-moving objects, we use *smooth* eye movements. However, when tracking fast-moving objects, we use *saccades*. Although everyone switches from smooth tracking to saccades as speed increases, some people are not unduly affected by increasing speed while others are. We say that some individuals are *velocity resistant*, while others are *velocity susceptible*.

Individual differences

Information Processing theorists claim that differences in the quality of perceptual skill is dependent on an interaction between abilities and learning. It is generally thought that abilities will only have a major effect on perception if they are in some way poorly developed. For example, we stated earlier that the ability to hear different levels of contact made by a table tennis bat on the ball helps the person to detect the amount of spin. If a person has sub-normal hearing their ability to perceive changes will be affected. However, if a person is within the normal range, the key factor becomes experience rather than ability. In other words, having above normal auditory ability does not a mean that your perception of what you hear will be better than a person with normal hearing.

One of the interesting phenomena, with regard to individual differences in perceptual performance that has been examined by cognitive psychologists, is the notion of perceptual styles. There are many theories concerning perceptual styles. All are continuum theories, i.e., they claim that individuals differ, in the way in which they attempt to deal with perceptual problems, along a continuum from one extreme to the other. Most people fall in the centre of the continuum.

Although there are many perceptual style theories, we will deal only with three here, as many of the theories have little bearing on sport and are more concerned with developmental issues than differences among adults. The first continuum which we will briefly examine is the *augmenters–reducers* continuum. Augmenters tend to exaggerate differences, e.g., distances between objects are perceived as being greater than they really are. Reducers, on the other hand, fail to perceive all of the information available in the environment, as a result they will perceive the distance between objects as being less than it really is. From this we can see that being at either end of the continuum can be detrimental to perceptual performance. It may, however, be an advantage in sports like boxing, American Football and Rugby to be a reducer, as you are likely to reduce the perception of pain caused by physical contact.

The second theory of perceptual style that we will look at is the *intuitive–plastic–analytic* continuum. At one end are individuals who make perceptual judgements intuitively. They appear to take in comparatively little information before making a judgement. As a result, decisions are made quickly but often inaccurately. At the other end of the continuum are analytical persons. These people examine all the possibilities before deciding on the nature of a display. They are much slower in making a judgement but generally more accurate. Individuals with a plastic perceptual style are ones who can alter their mode of perception to suit the problem. In situations that demand a quick decision, e.g., in many fast ball games, they will rely on intuition. While in situations in which there is plenty of time and where accuracy is important, e.g., climbing a mountain, they will be analytic.

The intuitive–plastic–analytic perceptual style has a great deal in common with Herman Witkin's (1950) *Field Dependence/Independence* theory. While very little research has been taken into the effect of the augmenter–reducer and intuitive–plastic–analytic styles on sports performance, the literature is full of experimental reports on the effect of Field Dependence/Independence. The differences in the ways that Field Dependent and Field Independent individuals process perceptual information is shown in Table 2.1. Those falling in the centre of the continuum are able to utilize both styles, although they can have problems using the Field Independent style if the problems are difficult to solve.

The characteristics of Field Independent people would appear to be advantageous to sports performance, especially in sports where there are complex displays to perceive. However, despite the fact that in many motor learning

Table 2.1 Characteristics of Field Dependent and Field Independent individuals (based on Witkin and Goodenough, 1980)

Field Dependent	Field Independent
Have difficulty in disembedding objects from their background	Have relative ease in disembedding objects from their background
Solve problems intuitively	Solve problems analytically
Are dominated by the present display	Can utilize cognitive restructuring skills (can picture ways in which the display can be changed)
Have difficulty in utilizing visuo-vestibular cue articulation; are either dominated by the visual or become confused	Have relative ease in utilizing visuo-vestibular cue articulation

texts you will see it stated that Field Independent individuals perform better than Field Dependent, the research literature does not fully support this. In fact, research results tend to be equivocal, i.e., some studies show an advantage for Field Independent participants, some an advantage for Field Dependent people and some no advantage for either. The main reasons that have been put forward for this are that there are differences in the nature of perceptual problems between those seen in sport and those in the tests of Field Dependence/Independence.

Field Dependence/Independence can be determined using various embedded figures tests (see Witkin *et al.*, 1970). It has been argued that the embedded figures test problems are far more complex than perceptual problems found in sport and there is more time allowed to solve them than a sports performer has available to him/her. Another factor that has been discussed is the fact that the embedded figures test is static while perception in sport takes place in a dynamic environment. It may also be that perceptual displays in sport do not include displays that are really 'embedding' displays. Witkin claimed that the Field Independent person only has an advantage over the Field Dependent if the environment is an embedding one. What he means by embedding is when the key factors are hidden within the display and are not immediately obvious.

It should be noted that the little research that has examined the effect of visuo-vestibular cue articulation on skills that require perception of how the body is oriented in space, e.g., gymnastics and trampolining, has shown unequivocally that being Field Independent is an advantage. Visuo-vestibular cue articulation is not tested by the embedded figures test but rather the rod-

and-frame test. (In this test, the person's visual field (the frame) is disrupted, so that spatial orientation is difficult. The task is to place the rod vertically, ignoring the confusing visual information, which 'encourages' the individual to place it at an angle off vertical.) These findings are probably due to the similarity between the demands of the skills and the rod-and–frame test.

Although sports require the individual to be intuitive at times and analytic at times, no research has, so far, been carried out examining the ability of individuals in the centre of the Field Dependent/Independent continuum compared to those at the two extremes. The failure to do this is also surprising given the fact that, in sport, some displays are embedded, in Witkin's meaning of the word, and some displays are not.

What is not clear with regard to individual differences is why and how they occur. Some factors are developmental, e.g., we move towards the Field Independent end of the continuum throughout childhood. Some differences would appear to be cultural, dependent on nurture more than nature. However, why individuals from the same culture should differ is difficult to explain.

Summary

From an Information Processing viewpoint, perception is indirect or inferred. It is dependent mainly on experience, although innate abilities will have some effect. Memory plays a large role in the way in which we solve perceptual problems, as does perceptual style. The key issues would appear to be selective attention and how we are able to attend to relevant stimuli while disregarding irrelevant ones.

Ecological psychology and perception

To the Information Processing theorists, perception precedes action and the two are separate. To the ecological psychologists, perception does not end *before* action is undertaken, it *continues* to be activated in order to control the movement. This is part of what the ecological psychologists call perception–action coupling, but it is only part of it. The other part is that perception itself is not carried out in isolation from action. *Action is necessary for perception to take place.* Gibson (1979) argued that *we perceive to act, and act to perceive*. In this section, we are concerned with the perception–action coupling which affects the initial perception of affordances. In Chapter 5, we examine the perception–action coupling affecting our ability to anticipate. While in Chapter 7, we look at the interaction with regard to motor control.

According to Gibson, perception is only possible if we *actively* search for affordances. A good example of this would be the research of Allard and colleagues (1980), outlined in the previous section. The basketball and volley-ball players in Allard's studies were visually searching the display for opportunities to act. The active nature of their search is demonstrated by the fact that all particpants, novice as well as expert, examined several parts of the display, they did not merely wait for the information to manifest itself.

The design used by Allard *et al.* meant that the participants had only to move their eyes in order to search for affordances. In real basketball and volleyball games, the players need to move their heads, as well as their eyes, to search the display effectively. These movements, the eyes in Allard's studies and the head and eyes in a real game, are examples of how action affects perception. *Without this movement, perception cannot take place.*

In order to visually perceive an affordance, an individual may need to include movement of far more than his/her head and eyes. Take the example of a golfer, whose approach to the green is blocked by a tree. The golfer will not only move eyes and head in order to examine all the possibilities, but will also move his/her whole body in order to view the problem from several different perspectives. Only then will the golfer perceive what affordances are available.

Moreover, each individual will perceive different affordances *from the same environment*. What an environment allows the individual to do will be dependent on the person's skills and abilities, as well as the layout of the display. A few years ago, I observed Alan Cunningham, a former Harlem Globetrotter, teaching a basketball class. At the end of the lesson, he bent down and picked the basketball up in one hand with his fingers pointing downwards. One of the class members also picked a ball up one handed, but placed his hand under the ball and balanced it on the top of his hand. As there was a massive difference between the span of the two individuals' hands, how they perceived the environment had to be different. To Cunningham, there was an affordance to pick the ball up fingers pointing downwards. To the student, the affordance was different.

I chose this example as it illustrates another key point in the ecological psychologists' theory of perception. The class member did not need to have past experience, of trying to pick up basketballs, to realise that he could not do the same as Cunningham. It was obvious from the size of the ball and the size of the person's hand that he was not able to pick it up one handed, with fingers pointing downwards. He could, however, see that he could balance it on his hand. *He did not need recourse to memory; all of the necessary information was present in the display.* This is what the ecological psychologists call *direct* perception.

Many students have difficulty in understanding the notion of direct perception, due to the fact that humans put labels on objects. While typing this manuscript, I am sitting on an ordinary chair. According to the ecological psychologists, I did not need to know that it is a chair in order to know that I can sit on it. When I entered the room my goal was to sit on something while typing. Given my knowledge of my own abilities, when I saw the chair I knew that I could sit on it. You may say, 'that is obvious, that is what chairs are for – sitting on'. If, however, I had never seen a chair before would I still have known that I could sit on it? To the ecological psychologists, the answer is a resounding 'yes'. Moreover, I can directly perceive that I can stand on the chair – I sometimes do when I wish to change a light bulb. Or I can kneel on it.

The ecological psychologist Michael Turvey (Turvey *et al.*, 1981) explains my perception as being that the chair is 'a sit on-able thing', 'a stand on-able thing' or 'a kneel on-able thing'. I do not need to know that it is called a chair to know that I can do these things. To a baby, however, the chair may only be 'a sit on-able thing' if placed on the chair by an adult. To a baby, who is just learning to stand, the chair may represent 'a climb up-able thing' and 'a lean on-able thing'. I have used the example of the baby for two reasons. Firstly, to show that the same object provides different affordances for myself and the baby because of our different sizes and abilities. Secondly, although I know what a chair is and have seen it used for many different things – in the cowboy films of my childhood it was 'a smash-able over the head thing' – the baby does not know what it is called and has no (or very limited) past experience of it. To explain this in a sporting context, we can try to use Turvey's method of describing what we perceive to explain the affordances of different sports equipment. A ball is a 'kickable thing', a 'headable thing', a 'catchable thing', while a hockey stick is a 'thing to hit with', a 'thing to dribble with' and a 'thing to stop a ball with'.

So far in this section, we have been discussing simple objects but in the section on perception and Information Processing Theory we examined the perception of complex displays. To the Information Processing theorist, the perception of such displays is heavily dependent on memory. To the ecological psychologists, even the complex displays found in team games, like soccer, Rugby and hockey, provide sufficient direct information to make recourse to memory unnecessary. As long as we know what our goal is and we know our own abilities, we will be able to recognize what the display affords. When a Rugby player receives the ball, he/she will search the display to see if it is possible to run over the opposition try line. Soccer or hockey players receiving the ball, near to the opposition goal, will look to see if they can shoot. Past experience is not necessary. Ecological psychologists accept that this search can be very time consuming – too time consuming in sport – if every affordance has to be examined. They claim that we overcome this by becoming *attuned to the affordances* that the environment offers. In other words, once we become attuned to the affordance, we will automatically search the part of the display that is most likely to provide us with the opportunity to achieve our goal. For example, a soccer centre-forward, who receives the ball in the opposition's penalty area, will look for chances to shoot.

The decision as to which areas of the display to search is similar to what the Information Processing theorists call selective attention. Similarly, the ecological psychologists, like the Information Processing theorists, claim that some information stands out more readily than other cues or affordances. We examined this with regards to Signal Detection Theory. Indeed, Signal Detection Theory would be almost totally acceptable to ecological psychologists.

Ecological psychologists differ from Information Processing theorists, however, on the nature and role of the senses. While Information Processing theorists see the senses as a means towards perception, the ecological psychologists see the senses as an integral part of perception. Perception begins with the act of searching the environment and the information picked up by this search is *meaningful* to the senses. That is, the information is not a series of nerve impulses or light waves that need to be processed by the CNS; it is meaningful information in its own right. If I search a display for a ball, I do not see light waves then determine that these are a ball because I have seen a ball previously. What I perceive is a 'kick-able thing', 'a throw-able thing' or 'a catch-able thing'. Moreover, I perceive not only a ball but a ball that is 'doing' something. My perception of a static ball is different from my perception of a ball coming towards me, which in turn is different from my perception of a ball going away from me. This, however, leaves the question: how can I perceive these different situations without recourse to memory?

According to the ecological psychologists, direct perception (no recourse to memory) is possible because, as we develop during early childhood, we become aware of the rules of nature and through these we are able to make sense of the world around us. An example would be the way in which light rays follow certain laws. If we take the example of perceiving a ball, light waves *flow* from the person's eyes to the ball and from the ball to the person. If the ball is static, the flow will remain the same; however, if the ball is moving, the flow will change and the person will be able to perceive motion. Moreover, the effect of changes in the flow will tell the individual where and how the ball is moving. The most obvious example of this is when a ball is coming towards us. As it gets nearer to us, its image gets bigger. The rate at which the size of the image increases will give us information about the speed of the ball.

Our ability to perceive that an object is coming towards us rather than increasing in size is because we take in information from the entire display. An object moving towards us gradually blocks out more and more of the environment. We can perceive relative change in relation to the display *behind and in front of* the object. What you can see between you and the object gets less and less. If the object was increasing in size, rather than coming towards us, it would block out more and more of the display behind itself but information *in front of* it would be unchanged (see Figure 2.6). This is similar to perceiving two objects in the distance. Both may appear to be the same size but the way in which they affect the display around themselves allows us to decide whether or not one is nearer to us or whether they are both the same distance away but of different actual sizes.

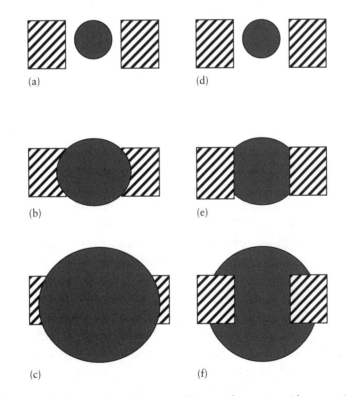

Figure 2.6 How the interaction between object and context aid perception: (a) to (c) represent how the display appears when the black object 'moves' towards the reader. (note the relationship with the two squares); (d) to (f) show what happens if the object stays in the same position but gets larger (again, note the relationship with the two squares)

Criticisms of the ecological approach

The major criticism of ecological psychology is the insistence that perception has no recourse to memory. Cognitivists have argued that sensory information cannot be made sense of without recourse to the CNS and in particular to working memory. While most ecological psychologists accept that we become more attuned to perceptual information with experience, they point to the fact that we can perceive adequately in novel situations as proof of the direct nature of perception. However, the explanation of how and why we become attuned to affordances is limited. Similarly, the way in which we become aware of the rules of nature, as we develop, is not explained.

Summary

According to the ecological psychologists, perception is direct and requires no recourse to memory. Perception begins when we search a display for information; therefore it is active and is coupled with action. The senses are part of the perceptual process. We directly perceive what an environment affords to us and do not require past experience of similar situations in order to make sense of the world around us.

Conclusion

Although there are many differences in the explanations of perception put forward by the Information Processing theorists and ecological psychologists, there are also many points of agreement. Indeed several authors have argued that, in many ways, the two schools are explaining the same phenomena but at different levels of processing. What the Information Processing theorists call selective attention, the ability to focus on relevant information, is very similar to the ecological psychologists claim that we search the environment for affordances. For example, both schools accept that visual search is an important factor in perception. Similarly, they accept that some information is easier to perceive than other information. Signal Detection Theory would be acceptable to both schools.

The major difference between the two schools is the role of memory. To the Information Processing theorists, perception is dependent on the efficiency of working memory. To the ecological psychologists, memory plays little or no part in perception and all the necessary information is present in the display. Undoubtedly, there is a major difference in the claims as to what role memory plays in perception, but the difference may not be as great as first thought.

Although the original ecological psychology theorists refused to accept any notion of mental representation, most of them now accept some form of representation – they would, however, balk at the use of the term 'memory'. Ecological psychologists agree that experience leads to a greater attunement to the affordances offered by an environment. To them, however, this attunement enables the person to search the areas of the display that contain the most relevant information. Once the area has been searched, the individual will directly perceive what the situation affords. They do not need to compare what they are seeing now with past experience in order to make sense of it.

Leaving aside theoretical differences, we need to end this section by stating what both schools agree happens when we perceive an environment. We undoubtedly need to know which areas of a display to examine and which to ignore. There is also no doubt that perception is necessary for action to take place. If we do not perceive accurately, we can not act correctly. There is, also, no doubt that perception becomes more efficient with experience. Whether this perception is direct or indirect is another matter. It is up to you to decide which school you accept as being correct. From a personal point of view, I believe that we can only make sense of some situations if we compare what we are seeing or feeling with similar situations that we have encountered in the past. In other situations, however, there is no need for recourse to memory. All the information is obviously present in the display. An example of the former would be observing a scrum in action in Rugby Union or the linemen in American Football. Without past experience, it is almost impossible to perceive what is happening. An example of the latter would be in a tennis game, where your opponent is in the right-hand side of the court, leaving the left-hand side open. If you know the rules of tennis, you do not need to have recourse to memory to see that this is an opportunity to play a passing shot.

Key points

Information Processing Theory and perception

- Information from the senses is in the form of nerve impulses, light waves, sound waves, etc. and, in it itself, does not make sense.

- Vision is the most important of the senses.

- There are two forms of vision:

  - foveal or focal (central vision, providing detailed information),

  - ambient vision (central and peripheral vision, supplying general information which is used to control posture, movement, etc.).

- Perception is indirect or inferred:

  - it requires organization, interpretation and integration of sensory information,

  - it is dependent on memory.

- Signal Detection Theory states that

  - signals must be perceived against a background of 'noise'.

- Detection is dependent on:

  - the strength of the stimulus in comparison to the noise,

  - the sensitivity of the individual, as measured by d-prime,

  - the individual's personal bias, as measured by the criterion C (how important detection is to the individual).

- The person may commit errors of:

  - omission (missing signals when they are present),

  - commission (perceiving signals that are not there),

  - omission occurs when the criterion is too low or too great,

  - commission only occurs when the criterion is too great.

- Pattern recognition is the ability to recognize a signal when only partial information is available.

- Selective attention is the ability to focus on relevant information and ignore irrelevant cues.

- Selective attention is necessary because we have a limited channel capacity.

- The main theories concerning channel capacity are:

  - single-channel theory (we can only deal with one thing at a time),

  - multi-channel theory (we have several channels, each responsible for different processes, plus a superordinate channel responsible for cognition),

  - fixed channel capacity theories (we have a limited capacity that does not change),

  - flexible channel capacity theories (we have a limited capacity but it can change depending on the situation, e.g., increases in arousal lead to increased capacity),

  - allocatable resources theories (attention is dependent on where we focus attention, this is the role of cognitive effort).

- The main theories of how we block out irrelevant information are:

  - Broadbent's filter theory (irrelevant information is filtered out in the short-term memory),

  - Treisman's theory (irrelevant information is 'attenuated' rather than discarded and is still processed, if familiar),

  - Norman's theory (the same as Treisman's except that 'pertinent' information is processed as well as the chosen stimuli).

- Visual search aids selective attention by searching the environment for relevant cues.

- Visual search can be aided by perceptual abilities such as:

  o span of apprehension (all the information that can be perceived in one glance),

  o vertical peripheral vision (especially dynamic vision),

  o horizontal peripheral vision (especially dynamic vision),

  o dynamic visual acuity (the ability to perceive moving objects).

- Individuals are thought to possess different perceptual styles, these are continuum theories.

- Examples of perceptual styles are:

  o augmenters (exaggerate differences) versus reducers (underrate differences),

  o intuitive (take in little information before making a decision; can be quick but inaccurate) versus plastic (can operate intuitively or analytically depending on the situation) versus analytic (take in a great deal of information before making a decision; can be slow and ponderous),

  o Field Dependent (have difficulty in disembedding objects from the background, act intuitively, are dominated by the current visual display, cannot articulate visual and vestibular information) versus Field Independent (are relatively good at disembedding information from the background, are analytic, can picture what a display would look like if it were to change, can articulate visual and vestibular information).

Ecological psychology and perception

- Perception is direct:

  o it does not require past experience,

  o all the necessary information is present in the environment.

- Perception is active (we must search the environment):

- we must act in order to perceive, therefore perception is a part of action: perception–action coupling,

- we search the environment for affordances (what the environment allows us to do).

- The same environment will offer different affordances to different people, depending on their physical, mental and emotional make-up.

- We do not need to label objects to know what we can do with them (a ball is not a 'ball', it is a 'kick-able thing' or a 'catch-able thing').

- With exposure to environments, we become attuned to the affordances they offer (i.e., we know where in the environment to search for the affordance).

Test your knowledge

(Answers in Appendix 3.)

Part one

Choose which of the phrases, (a), (b), (c) or (d), is the most accurate. There is only *one* correct answer for each problem.

1　The normal range of foveal vision is:

    (a) 1°–4°,

    (b) 2°–5°,

    (c) 3°–6°,

    (d) 4°–8°.

2.　According to Information Processing Theory, the senses:

    (a) integrate incoming information,

    (b) organize incoming information,

    (c) relay meaningful information to the CNS,

(d) relay meaningless information to the CNS.

3. According to Signal Detection Theory, which of the following ball/background combinations would best aid detection of the ball?

(a) light blue ball/light green background,

(b) yellow ball/maroon background,

(c) red ball/green background,

(d) white ball/light green background.

4. According to Signal Detection Theory, the under-aroused individual may commit errors of:

(a) commission,

(b) omission,

(c) omission and commission,

(d) stimulus rejection.

5. The ability to detect a signal when only partial information is available is called:

(a) pattern recognition,

(b) signal detection,

(c) selective attention,

(d) noise rejection.

6. Research into dual-task performance has shown that:

(a) tasks using different CNS pathways can be carried out simultaneously without interference,

(b) tasks using similar CNS pathways can be carried out simultaneously without interference,

(c) even well-learned automatic skills are affected by simultaneous performance,

(d) a well-learned task is only affected by dual performance if the other task is novel.

7. Broadbent, Treisman and Norman developed theories of selective attention, *all* of which emphasize:

   (a) the attenuation of information,

   (b) the pertinence of information,

   (c) the selective filter,

   (d) cognitive effort.

8. Allard, Graham and Paarsalu (1980) and Allard and Starkes (1980) showed that expert basketball and volleyball players searched firstly for:

   (a) where their team-mates were positioned,

   (b) where their opponents were positioned,

   (c) spaces between opponents,

   (d) spaces behind defenders.

9. Allard, Graham and Paarsalu (1980) and Allard and Starkes (1980) showed that inexperienced basketball and volleyball players searched firstly for:

   (a) where their team-mates were positioned,

   (b) where their opponents were positioned,

   (c) spaces between opponents,

   (d) spaces behind defenders.

10. Which of the following is the most important factor in aiding sports performance?

   (a) static visual acuity,

   (b) static depth perception,

   (c) dynamic visual acuity,

(d) static and dynamic depth perception.

11. Field Dependent individuals:

   (a) act intuitively,

   (b) are analytical,

   (c) minimize differences,

   (d) accentuate differences.

12. Field Independent individuals have been shown to have an advantage over Field Dependent persons in tasks such as:

   (a) swimming,

   (b) diving,

   (c) dodging,

   (d) hopping.

13. Reducers probably have an advantage over augmenters in:

   (a) climbing,

   (b) archery,

   (c) shooting,

   (d) boxing.

14. According to Action Systems Theory, perception improves with experience due to:

   (a) an increase in long-term memory stores,

   (b) the development of neural engrams in the CNS,

   (c) greater sensitivity to the presence of affordances,

   (d) greater awareness of functional specificity.

15. According to Action Systems Theory, sensation:

   (a) provides meaningless information to the CNS,

(b) precedes action,

(c) is an integral part of perception,

(d) aids memory.

Part two

Fill in the blank spaces using words taken from the list below (NB there are more words in the list than there are spaces).

1. There are two types of vision, _____ and _____.

2. _____ can help table tennis players to know the amount of spin that has been placed on the ball.

3. According to Information Processing Theory, _____ is inferred or _____.

4. According to Information Processing Theory, perception is the organization, _____ and _____ of sensory _____.

5. Swets (1964), in his Signal Detection Theory, stated that detection of a signal would be affected by the _____ of the signal compared with the _____ of the background noise.

6. In Signal Detection Theory, d-prime represents the individual's _____.

7. In Signal Detection Theory, the criterion represents the individual's _____.

8. In tennis, pattern recognition allows us to _____ what shot our opponent is going to play before he/she has hit the ball.

9. When we see an object moving towards us, then lose sight of it, we are still able to 'know' the trajectory of the object because of the phenomenon called _____.

10. We need _____ _____ because we are limited in the amount of information with which we can deal at any one time.

11. With regard to CNS capacity, Deutsch and Deutsch (1963) claimed that capacity was _____, while Kahneman (1973) stated that it was _____.

12. According to Kahneman (1973), cognitive effort is responsible for the _____ of _____.

13. According to Norman (1969), we process information that is _____.

14. Individuals whose perception of objects is negatively affected by movement are said to be _____ _____.

15. The amount of information we can perceive in one glance is called the span of _____.

16. We visually track fast-moving objects using _____.

17. The _____ – _____ –analytic continuum is a theory of perceptual style.

18. According to Action Systems Theory, _____ is necessary for perception to take place.

19. To the ecological psychologists, all the information that we need is present in the display, we do not need _____.

20. Ecological psychologists use the term _____ to describe what the environment allows us to do.

21. Experience allows us to become _____ to affordances.

22. According to Dynamical Systems Theory, information in the environment is _____ and does not have to be processed by the CNS.

integration	velocity	strength	attention	ambient	affordance
plastic	perception	bias	flexible	audition	indirect
resources	foveal	intuitive	interpretation	sensitivity	intensity
information	meaningful	fixed	susceptible	apprehension	selective
allocation	pertinent	closure	attuned	saccades	direct
noise	action	memory	anticipate		

Additional reading

Abernethy B (1987) Review: selective attention in fast ball sports. I: General principles. *Australian J Sci Med Sport* **19**: 3–6

Abernethy B (1987) Review: selective attention in fast ball sports. II: Expert–novice differences. *Australian J Sci Med Sport* **19**: 7–15

Wrisberg CA (2000) Sensory contributions to skilled performance. In: *Study guide to motor learning and performance*, Wrisberg CA (Ed) Human Kinetics, Champaign, Illinois, USA, pp. 39–52

3 Decision Making

Learning Objectives

By the end of the chapter, you should be able to

♦ understand what is meant by decision making during skilled performance

♦ understand the importance of decision making in skilled performance

♦ understand the role of working memory in decision making

♦ understand the difference between declarative and procedural knowledge

♦ understand how individual differences affect decision-making performance

♦ understand the problems of carrying out research into decision making

Acquisition and Performance of Sports Skills   T. McMorris
© 2004 John Wiley & Sons, Ltd   ISBNs: 0-470-84994-0 (HB); 0-470-84995-9 (PB)

Introduction

To the Information Processing theorists, decision making follows perception and precedes action. It is vital if a skilled performance is going to take place. The ecological psychologists tend not to use the term 'decision making'. Several authors have stated that ecological psychology is not concerned with decision making at all, and it is the preserve of the cognitivists. While I accept that most research and writing on the subject has come from an Information Processing perspective, I do not agree that ecological psychology does not cover this area. I do, however, accept that what the Information Processing theorists call decision making is seen by the ecological psychologists as being that part of perception–action coupling which allows us to achieve our goal. We will deal with this later in the chapter.

Information Processing Theory and decision making

To the cognitivists, the decision-making part of the Information Processing model explains *how we use perception and past experience to determine what action to take in any given situation*. The ability to know what to do in different situations, during sports performance, is essential. Sport is full of examples of performers who have limited innate abilities yet are able to play at the top level due to their ability to utilize their strengths and hide their weaknesses. One of the most obvious examples, to me, is Bobby Moore, who captained England to their World Cup win in 1966. Moore is generally accepted as being one of the best defenders ever to have played soccer. He was, however, only average height, a rather slow runner and of only average strength. If we examined Moore's abilities, he would look to be a very ordinary physical specimen. However, he rarely made an error in decision making. He made up for his lack of physical skills by *doing the right thing, at the right time*. Another example is Wayne Gretsky, arguably the greatest ice hockey player ever. Gretsky had very good stick handling skill but, in a very physical game, he appeared to lack the necessary speed and physique. Like Moore, he made up for this by his excellent decision making. Perhaps the most striking example of all is Tyronne Bogues, who played basketball in the NBA despite being only 1.6 m (5 ft 3 inches) tall.

In the above paragraph, I italicized 'doing the right thing at the right time'. This is because basically that is what we mean when we say that someone has good decision-making ability. Another term that we often hear used is to say that someone is 'a good reader of the game'. While these 'definitions' may be fine, they lack a great deal of precision. Therefore, I prefer Barbara Knapp's definition. She wrote that decision making is *'knowing which technique to use in any given situation'* (Knapp, 1963). Having good technique means having the ability to carry out the *motor* aspect of the task. The whole skill is demonstrated by *technique plus decision making*. The greater the range of techniques a person has, the better equipped they are to perform well. However, if they use the wrong technique at the wrong time, their 'skill' is poor. On the other hand, players with limited techniques can perform skilfully by using what ability they have at the correct time.

According to Information Processing Theory, the ability to make accurate decisions is a complex affair. Examining the Information Processing model (Figure 1.4) we can see that the input is interpreted at the perception stage and the chosen cues are passed to the STM, where they are compared to past experience recalled from the LTM. Based on this comparison a decision as to what to do is made. Baddeley (1986) called this process *working memory*. More recent cognitive models have attempted to explain the process but they differ very little from Baddeley's ideas.

When we look at the explanation of working memory above, it appears that decision making is a fairly simple task. However, when we look more closely we can see the problems. Perception must be accurate if good decisions are to be made. If the wrong information is passed to the STM, a wrong decision is inevitable. Selective attention allows us to ensure that we perceive the correct information and pass it to the STM. It may appear to some of you that comparing the information passed to the STM with past experience held in the LTM is a simple affair. This is far from the case because no two situations are ever identical. It is naïve to say (as the very early Information Processing theorists did) that we examine the present display, recall what we did last time in such a display, and repeat any successful actions. More recent theories, such as Schmidt's (1975) Schema Theory (see Chapter 8), state that we do not try to recall specific and precise past situations but rather generalized rules or schemas. These allow us to make an accurate decision regardless of differences between the present situation and past experiences. Although this is a better explanation than earlier theories, Information Processing Theory is still unable to explain how we can perform in novel situations for which we have no schemas.

Another problem with the Information Processing theorists' explanation of how we make decisions is that the amount of information that must be held in the STM and recalled from the LTM, in order to make a good decision, is immense. Comparing the information must be time consuming, yet we see sports performers make extremely quick decisions in very complex environments. Information Processing Theory does not adequately explain how we are able to make decisions as quickly as we do. One explanation is that we semi-prepare the decision before we perform. The most widely quoted theory explaining this phenomenon is that of Anderson (1982).

Anderson's *Adaptive Control of Thought (ACT)* theory states that we *predetermine* what we will do in any given situation. Anderson claims that we go through a series of *'if this happens, then we do that'* decisions. The decision is still based on past experience but deciding beforehand, what we will do, allows us to respond quickly. This is often necessary in team games. Indeed in many American sports, e.g., American Football and basketball, the plays may be called by the coach and the players simply do what was previously practised. This is very like the training in the military, where combatants practice set responses over and over again until they become automatic. Anderson has revised his original theory (Anderson and Lebiere, 1998), but the changes are small and the original version is still referred to in sports psychology.

Automatic responses are not always possible and players are often left to make decisions 'on the spot'. A number of authors, myself included, have argued that we are able to do this because we follow a hierarchical response pattern. An example of such a hierarchy is provided in Figure 3.1. Since advocating the hierarchical response explanation, I have become somewhat dubious of its validity. I admit that, in many sports, players practice going through a series of hierarchical responses similar to those in Figure 3.1. Indeed my own hierarchies are based on the principles of play in soccer and on what I was taught on Football Association coaching courses. However, it now appears to me, that going through such hierarchies is too onerous and ponderous. I believe that these hierarchies help us to decide what is the best option in any given situation, while learning. Once we have learnt, we switch into an 'if this happens then we do that' mode, as Anderson suggests.

According to ACT, the period of time when we learn what to do in any given situation is said to be the time taken to develop *declarative knowledge*. Declarative knowledge is knowing *what* to do. Anderson believes that we acquire declarative knowledge prior to what he terms *procedural knowledge*. Procedural knowledge is not merely making the correct decision but knowing how to ensure that the goal of our action is met. It is difficult to argue against a claim that there is a difference between knowing what to do and being able to do it. Many coaches are very good at the former but were not as good as their athletes at the latter. There is, however, no proof that declarative knowledge precedes procedural knowledge in sport. Research carried out by Mark Williams, Keith Davids and colleagues (e.g., Williams and Davids, 1995) has

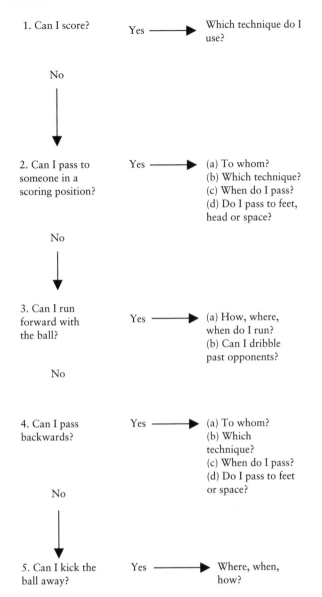

Figure 3.1   Hierarchy of options open to a soccer player when making decisions while attacking (from McMorris, 1986)

shown unequivocally that expert performers have greater declarative knowledge, as well as procedural knowledge, than intermediate and novice performers. As they themselves point out, this does not prove that declarative knowledge precedes procedural knowledge. It may well be that greater exposure to the sport means that the expert has picked up more declarative knowledge. They may not, however, use this when acquiring procedural knowledge.

This was highlighted to me many years ago when attending a Football Association coaching course. The coach in charge wanted to show how to dribble past a defender. One of the people on the course was Wilf Mannion, a former England international. The coach gave Mannion, then aged about 55, the ball and told him to dribble past a young professional player. It seemed a crazy thing to ask a comparatively old man to beat a young professional. Nevertheless, Mannion left the youngster beaten several times. The coach then brought in a covering defender and asked Mannion to dribble the two of them. Mannion shuffled up to the two young players, his eyes on the covering player. The defenders did well, at first, but the covering player came too close to the first defender for a split second. That was all Mannion needed and he went past the two of them. The coach then asked Mannion to explain what he had done – he could not. I knew what he had done, but although I was about 25 years younger than Mannion, I would not have been able to go past the two professional defenders. This example, also, says much about how easy it is to overestimate the ageing process; two very embarrassed young professionals went home that night. We will return to declarative and procedural knowledge in Chapter 8 when discussing learning.

Individual differences

Apart from expert–novice differences and, to a lesser extent, expert–intermediate player differences, little research has examined why and how individuals differ in their ability to make decisions. A number of authors have compared the ability of individuals possessing Field Dependent and Field Independent cognitive styles. As you no doubt remember from the previous chapter, Field Independent people are categorized by the ability to disembed objects from the background, solve problems analytically and utilize cognitive restructuring skills, i.e., picture what the present display will look like if they or other players move. Field Dependent individuals have comparative difficulty in disembedding objects from their background, solve problems intuitively and their perception is dominated by the present display. One would assume that Field Independent individuals would have a clear advantage over Field Dependent in decision making, but this has not been borne out by research. It would appear that there is no difference. The reasons for the failure to demonstrate a difference may be similar to those I outlined in the last chapter, concerning the affect of Field Dependence/Independence on perception. Moreover, it does not appear that the problems facing the decision-maker, in sport, are sufficiently complex to make being Field Independent an advantage.

Another factor that might affect decision making is age. Research examining age group differences has, however, shown that the older age groups are better than the younger, only if there is a gap between the two groups of at least 2 years. In fact, some research has only shown significant differences when the age difference is of 4 or more years. This is not as strange as it may first appear. According to Piagetian and neo-Piagetian theories of cognitive development, children move from one sub-stage to another about every 2 years. Therefore, improvement appears to be dependent on such a change.

It would seem that, in adults, the only individual factor to make a significant difference is experience. This supports the claims of Information Processing theorists that the key factor is the person's LTM store. The greater the store, the easier it is to 'call up' experiences from LTM, to be compared with information held in the STM.

Dynamical Systems Theory and goal achievement

I was tempted to call this section 'Dynamical Systems Theory and decision making'. However, Dynamical Systems theorists do not talk about decision making, as such. They are concerned with goal setting and what actions the environment allows the player to make in order to achieve his/her goal. According to Dynamical Systems Theory, the role of the CNS is to determine the goals of any action to be taken. This will depend on the *constraints* placed before the individual. These constraints will be *task, organismic* and *environmental*.

The rules of the game are task constraints. In tennis, for example, the rules will force the individual to search for opportunities to hit the ball past their opponent. The principles of play will also affect the affordances that the person searches for. In field hockey, if the individual knows that ball possession is one of the goals of the game, he/she will look for opportunities to pass to a team-mate. The organismic constraints are the limitations that the individuals themselves bring to the activity – how strong they are, or how fast, or how tall. Thus different people will do different things in the same situation. The NBA players Earl Boykins and Shawn Bradley highlight this. With a height of 1.7 m (5 ft 6 inches) Boykins must take up different positions on the basketball court, if he wants to receive a pass, compared with the 2.3 m (7 ft 6 inches) Bradley. The environmental constraints are such factors as the weather and the size of the playing area. For example, the correct decision when playing Rugby on a firm surface will be very different to that when playing in mud.

Once the person has determined what opportunities to search for, the environment supplies all the necessary information. The individual can perceive gaps between and behind defenders, opportunities to shoot at goal or basket, or whether a defender is fast or slow. Given that the player knows what he/she wishes to do, they will automatically react when the opportunity to achieve the goal presents itself.

Although the Dynamical Systems theorists deny the role of memory, they do accept that experience is important. Without experience the person will not be able to set the correct goals and will not recognize affordances when they occur. Experience helps us to know which parts of the environment are the most likely to offer opportunities to achieve our goal. Therefore, we search these areas. We do not need to use memory to either process the affordance or decide what action to take. The environment will dictate what we can do and not do. For example, a basketball player will examine spaces behind and between defenders that might offer the affordance to drive for the basket. If the affordance is there, they will drive in. They do not need to say 'last time I saw this situation, I chose to drive for basket'. They simply know what to do because it is obvious.

Research findings and problems with research design

The fact that very little research has been undertaken into decision making in sport may be due to difficulties with the mechanics of producing valid and reliable tests of decision making. Following the example of Charles Thiffault (1980), several researchers have used tachistoscopically presented tests. Thiffault's test examined the decision-making ability of ice hockey players, but most other research has looked at ball games. In these tests, slides of typical game situations are produced and shown to the participants on a slide projector fitted with a tachistoscopic timing device. The participant is asked to make a decision, normally for the player in possession of the ball, as to what action should be taken. The decision has to be made as accurately and as quickly as possible.

The major problem with such tests is that the display is static, whereas in real-life situations the display is dynamic. In order to overcome this criticism, Helsen and Pauwels (1988) developed video-based tests. Helsen and Pauwels showed participants video clips of soccer games and 'froze' the action at chosen times. This is when the decision had to be made. Furthermore, Helsen and Pauwels had the participants stand facing a screen with a soccer ball at their feet and asked them to pass, shoot or run with the ball dependent on what action they thought the player should take. This is, of course, more realistic than simply stating what decision someone should make.

Other methods of examining decision-making performance have been used. Subjective assessment by experienced coaches has been favoured by some researchers. This method, however, needs to be controlled as much as possible. The coaches should be given guidelines to aid their assessment and more than one coach should be used wherever possible. Table 3.1 shows the guidelines that I developed for testing decision making in soccer. Some researchers have

Table 3.1 Guidelines for testing decision-making performance in soccer (from McMorris, 1986)

Rating	Description
5	Knows how, where and when to improvise and move forward
	Knows how, where and when to run in order to create space for others
	Can anticipate the opposition's play when defending
	Gives verbal information to other players
	Knows how to deal with two attackers
4	Knows when to pass the ball behind the defence
	Knows when and where to cover a defender who is pressurizing an attacker
	Knows when and how to move wide
	Knows how to 'check off' an opponent
3	Knows when, where and how to pass
	Knows when to control the ball and when to play it first time
	Knows when and where to support behind the ball
	Knows when to pass the ball forward, square and back
	Knows where and when to delay and tackle
	Knows when to balance the defence
	Knows how to make a recovery run and when to mark opponents
	Knows where and when to dribble and knows when to shoot
2	Makes wrong choice of when, how or where to pass
	Controls the ball in situations that demand first time play
	Makes wrong choice of when and where to support
	Does not balance the defence and does not know where to dribble
	Fails to perceive shooting opportunities
1	Makes wrong choice of when, how and where to pass
	Makes wrong choice of when and where to support
	Does not provide width and does not mark opponents

asked players to give running commentaries, during actual competition, on why they have chosen that particular action. This is similar to the Ministry of Transport advanced driving test. Other researchers, particularly those testing children, have given their participants pencil and paper tests. Figure 3.2 shows an example of this.

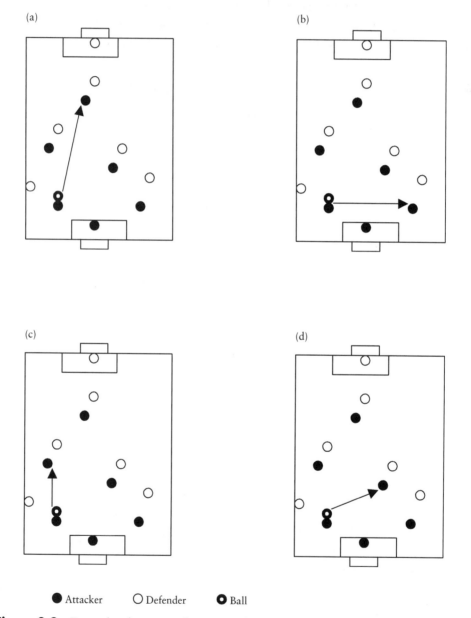

Figure 3.2 Example of a soccer decision-making task; the person must decide which is the correct option (a), (b), (c) or (d)

Although the tests differ the results are the same. Experts make decisions faster than novices and intermediate-level players. Experts are generally, though not always, more accurate than novices and intermediate performers, while the latter do better than novices. With children, the older children do better than the younger ones.

Conclusion

Both Information Processing and Dynamical Systems Theories assert the importance of good selective attention, the need to search the relevant parts of the display. To the Information Processing theorists, this allows the person to perceive the present display and to extract similar past experiences from LTM. To the Dynamical Systems theorists, it allows the individual to achieve his/her goal. Both theories accept that experience plays a major role in the choice of areas of the display to which they should attend. This emphasis on the importance of experience is borne out by research.

While Dynamical Systems Theory emphasizes the importance of task, organismic and environmental constraints on the making of decisions, this is not neglected by the Information Processing theorists. It is implicit within the comparison of present and past experience taking place in working memory. My colleague Bill MacGillivary and I, writing from an Information Processing approach, pointed out that in making a decision in soccer, the players would have to take account of their own strengths and weaknesses, the strengths and weaknesses of team-mates and opponents, the condition of the pitch, the weather and the score at that particular moment (McMorris and MacGillivary, 1988). These factors are no different from organismic (their own strengths and weaknesses, the strengths and weaknesses of team-mates and opponents), environmental (the condition of the pitch, the weather) and task (the score at that particular moment) constraints.

Implications for coaches and players

Despite the fact that making good decisions is vital to good performance, it is an area that is often neglected by coaches, teachers and players. Over a 3-year period from 1999 to 2002, I carried out an investigation into how many of my students had been taught decision making in school and at sports clubs. Less than 3 per cent had received any teaching in school and this rose only to just under 5 per cent for those playing in clubs. This neglect has been recognized for some time. Dave Bunker and Rod Thorpe (1982) initiated the Teaching Games for Understanding (TGFU) approach partly to eradicate this problem. This approach favours the teaching of decision making rather than techniques. While it should be noted that TGFU was primarily introduced for pedagogical reasons not related to performance but to the enjoyment of sport, it has heralded an acceptance among physical educationalists that decision making should be taught in schools. From my research, it does not look as though this is being carried out in practice.

While the reason for this may be because decision making is difficult to teach and requires a good knowledge of the activity, it may also be because teachers and coaches fail to understand its importance. When spectating our attention is drawn to the skilful performance of techniques. If we ask spectators what they admire most about Venus Williams, they might say the strength and accuracy of her volleys. What they are unlikely to say is how she manipulates play to allow her to use her volley. Thorpe and Bunker argued that we should educate future spectators to be aware of decision-making elements of performance, as it will aid their ability to enjoy spectating. It could also be claimed that it would make teachers and youth coaches aware of the need to teach decision making.

Key points

Information Processing Theory and decision making

- Decision making refers to the process by which we decide what action to take in any given situation:

    - Knapp (1963) referred to it as 'knowing which technique to use in any given situation'.

- Decision making is processed by working memory (perception–memory interaction).

- Decision making is very dependent on experience.

- According to Anderson we decide what we will do prior to taking part in an activity:

    o   we follow a series of predetermined responses (if 'a' happens, we will do 'b').

- Anderson believes that declarative knowledge (knowing what to do) needs to be acquired before procedural knowledge (knowing what to do and how to do it):

    o   there is no definitive proof that, in sport, declarative knowledge needs to be acquired before we can acquire procedural knowledge,

    o   procedural knowledge may be obtained subconsciously.

Dynamical Systems Theory and goal achievement

- We decide what we want to do in any given situation, and this will be determined by:

    o   task constraints (e.g., rules of the game),

    o   environmental constraints (what the environment allows or affords),

    o   organismic constraints (the strengths and weaknesses we bring to the task).

- We search the environment for affordances that allow us to achieve our goal:

    o   if we are attuned to the affordances, we will know which parts of the display to search.

Research designs

- The main research designs have been:

    o   tachistoscopic presentation of slides of game situations,

    o   video presentation of game situations.

- The main measures of performance have been:

- ○ accuracy of decision,

- ○ speed of response.

Research results

- Experienced players have generally been shown to be faster than inexperienced players.

- Experienced players are not always more accurate than inexperienced players.

Test your knowledge

(Answers in Appendix 3.)

Part one

Complete the following sentences using the phrases below.

1. Knapp (1963) defined decision making as _____ in any given situation.

2. Skill consists of _____.

3. Working memory consists of _____ and recall from long-term memory.

4. Schemas are _____.

5. Declarative knowledge is _____.

6. Procedural knowledge is _____.

7. According to Anderson's (1982) ACT Theory, we _____ in any given situation.

8. Field Independent people _____.

9. Field Dependent individuals _____.

10. According to Dynamical Systems Theory, the CNS _____.

11. The rules of a game are examples of _____.

perception, decision, short-term memory   determines the goals to be achieved
make decisions analytically   knowing what to do and how to do it
task constraints   generalized rules
predetermine what we will do   make decisions intuitively
decision making plus technique   knowing which technique to use
knowing what to do

Part two

Fill in the blank spaces using words from the list below (NB there are more words in the list than there are spaces).

1. To the Information Processing theorists, decision making is determined by our ability to use _____ and past experience.

2. It is possible to possess a large range of _____ and lack skill.

3. Schmidt (1975) claimed that we do not recall specific past experiences but _____ rules.

4. Anderson's (1982) ACT Theory explains how we are able to make decisions _____.

5. When learning to make decisions, we often follow a _____ of responses.

6. _____ knowledge is supposed to precede _____ knowledge, according to Anderson (1982).

7. According to Dynamical Systems Theory, two individuals will interact differently with the same environment because of their differing _____ constraints.

8. Weather conditions are an example of _____ constraints.

9. Once an affordance to achieve a goal has been perceived, _____ will take place automatically.

10. In research experiments, speed of decisions is measured using a _____ timing device.

11. Helsen and Pauwels' (1988) research design is better than previous designs because the way of measuring the decision is more _____.

12. For the subjective assessment of players' decision making to be effective, the assessors need _____.

13. Assessors also need to be _____.

14. Research has generally shown that experts make _____ decisions than novices.

15. Dynamical Systems theorists and Information Processing theorists agree that _____ helps the person to do make the correct move.

hierarchy	faster	environmental	realistic	procedural
action	experienced	quickly	guidelines	technique
tactics	generalized	organismic	tachistoscopic	
declarative	perception	experience		

Additional reading

Franks IM, Wilberg RB and Fishburne G (1982) Process of decision making: an application to team games. *Coaching Sci Update* **1982–83**: 12–16

Gréhaigne JF and Godbout P (1998) Formative assessment in team sports in a tactical approach context. *J Phys Ed, Rec Dance* **69**: 46–51

McMorris T and Graydon J (1997) The contribution of the research literature to the understanding of decision making in team games. *J Hum Movement Studies*, **33**: 69–90

Riley M and Roberton MA (1981) Developing skillful games players: consistency between beliefs and practice. *Motor Skills Theory into Practice* **5**: 123–133

4 Reaction Time

Learning Objectives

By the end of this chapter, you should be able to

- understand the nature of response time, reaction time and movement time

- understand the role of working memory in choice reaction time

- break reaction time down into its component parts

- understand the nature of the Hick–Hyman Law

- understand the role and effect of probability on choice reaction time

- understand the nature of the psychological refractory period

- understand how the following affect reaction time

  - ◊ arousal

  - ◊ stimulus intensity

  - ◊ stimulus familiarity

  - ◊ response complexity

  - ◊ sensory modality

  - ◊ psychological set

- understand the extent to which reaction time research supports Information Processing Theory

Acquisition and Performance of Sports Skills   T. McMorris
© 2004 John Wiley & Sons, Ltd   ISBNs: 0-470-84994-0 (HB); 0-470-84995-9 (PB)

Introduction

To the ecological psychologists, the study of reaction time is merely a matter of reporting what is observed. They are not concerned with trying to examine what is happening in the CNS, when we make fast responses. Therefore, this chapter takes an Information Processing Theory approach, only.

There is no doubt that the performance of many sports skills needs to be carried out very quickly, if the individual is to be successful. The batter in cricket facing a fast bowler, the tennis player receiving a serve or the goaltender in ice hockey trying to save a slap shot, all need to be able to respond quickly. It is also obvious that there are limitations in how quickly individuals can respond. Sometimes, what is required of us is beyond our capabilities.

Before examining how Information Processing Theory attempts to explain this, we need to be fully aware of what we mean by reaction time. The lay person often uses the term 'reaction time' when, in fact, they are talking about response time. *Response time* is the time from the *introduction of a stimulus to the completion of the action required to deal with the problem.* Figure 4.1 presents this diagrammatically. As you can see from Figure 4.1, response time is made up of reaction time and movement time. *Movement time* is the time it takes to carry out the motor aspects of the performance.

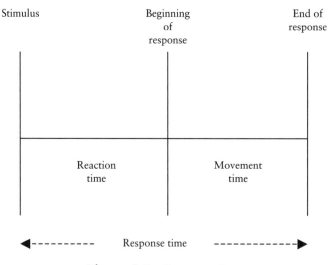

Figure 4.1   Response time

It should be noted that while reaction time and movement time will affect one another, they are separate entities. A person can have a fast reaction time but slow movement time or vice versa. Or someone can be quick or slow at both.

While movement time describes the overt physical activity, reaction time attempts to explain the covert CNS activity. *Reaction time is the time that elapses from the sudden onset of a stimulus to the beginning of an overt response* (Oxendine, 1968). The key point here is that, like response time, it starts with the introduction of the stimulus but ends at the *beginning* of the response, *before the motor act* begins.

Reaction time can be sub-divided into pre-motor time and motor time. *Pre-motor time* is the time from the onset of the stimulus to the transmission of the chosen motor action to the muscles. *Motor time* is the time it takes for the muscles to be activated by the efferent or motor nerves. Motor time is controlled by the PNS and differs very little between healthy individuals. Pre-motor time, however, can differ greatly between people. Pre-motor time is a product of both the CNS and PNS. It consists of the senses, transmission of the sensory information to the CNS, perception, decision making, efferent organization and transmission of the efferent information to the muscles. Thus we can see that it includes the entire Information Processing model, as shown in Figure 4.2.

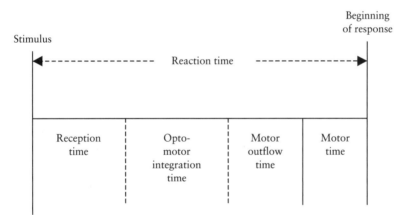

Figure 4.2 Reaction time (adapted from Kroll and Clarkson 1978); Reprinted, by permission, from W. Kroll and P.M. Clarkson, 1978, "Fractionated reflex time, resisted and unresisted fractionated time under normal and fatigued conditions" in *Psychology of motor behavior and sport – 1977*, edited by D.M. Landers and R.W. Christina (Champaign, IL: Human Kinetics), 110

Figure 4.2 shows a breakdown of reaction time. As we can see, pre-motor time is sub-divided into *reception time, opto-motor integration time* and *motor outflow time*. Reception time and motor outflow time, like motor time, are controlled by the PNS and differ very little between healthy individuals. On the other hand, opto-motor integration time can, and does, differ greatly between people. As you can see from Figure 4.2, opto-motor integration time is a product of working memory plus LTM and efferent organization. Thus, a study of reaction time allows us to examine the efficiency of how well we are able to process information.

One of the ways in which we can examine how we process information is to look at inter-individual differences in reaction time. However, reaction time does not only differ between people but it also demonstrates intra-individual differences, i.e., changes in reaction time within an individual from one situation to another. The purpose of the rest of this chapter is to examine these inter- and intra-individual differences.

Inter- and intra-individual differences

Although it is obvious, from the simple observation of different individuals performing skills, that people differ in the speed of their reactions, it is not easy to say why. The proficiency of working memory, the LTM store and the proficiency of efferent organization will all affect reaction time. However, most of the reasons for inter-individual differences are also reasons for intra-individual differences. For example, familiarity with a stimulus aids reaction time. Thus, as a person becomes more familiar with a stimulus their reaction time shortens. It is therefore tempting to say that if two people differ in their speed of reaction to a given stimulus, it is because one is more familiar with the stimulus than the other. This, however, ignores the fact that there are inter-individual differences in reaction time between individuals who have similar exposure to the stimulus. It would appear that inter-individual differences are genetic. As we saw in Chapter 1, reaction time is considered to be an ability and we are simply quick or we are not. As we will see below, when examining intra-individual differences, we can shorten our reaction time in several ways but we are still restricted by what we inherited from our parents.

One of the first factors to be examined that might affect intra-individual differences in reaction time was the interaction between the complexity of the stimulus or stimuli and the nature of the response or responses required. The first experiments in reaction time looked at what we call *simple reaction time*. Simple reaction time is when there is only one predetermined stimulus and the same response is required on each occasion. It is necessary for us to understand the basic findings of this research in order to understand reaction time in more complex situations. However, there are very few sports situations that fall into the category of simple reaction-time problems. The only ones I can think of are the start of track or swimming races.

The early reaction-time experiments required the participants to press a button as soon as they saw a light illuminated. The mean times for this ranged between 170 and 200 ms. However, the response required, pressing a button, is much more simple than starting a 100 m sprint, whether on land or in the water. We will look at how the difference in the required response affects the reaction time later in this section.

While the study of simple reaction time tells us little about sports performance, it also tells us little about the workings of the information-processing system. With simple reaction time there is no STM–LTM comparison, and the decision and efferent organization are predetermined. Moreover, the position of the stimulus is known, therefore the individual does not have to search for it. Although the early researchers were not concerned with sports performance, they were interested in finding out more about the information-processing system. Therefore, they decided to examine *choice reaction time.*

When examining choice reaction time, the early researchers used many different stimuli–response requirement protocols. To sports performers and coaches the most important are when there are several stimuli and a different response is needed for each stimulus. For visual choice reaction-time tests the normal set up is for the individual to sit facing a row of lights with buttons beneath each light. They are required to respond by pressing the button beneath whichever light is illuminated (see Figure 4.3). This condition places far greater stress on the information-processing system, and in particular opto-motor

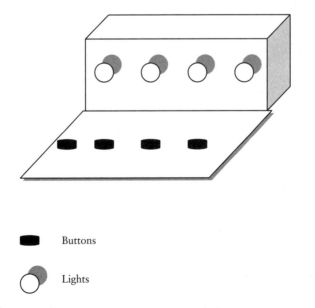

■ Buttons

◯ Lights

Figure 4.3   Diagram depicting a visual choice reaction timer

integration, than simple reaction time. It is therefore no surprise to find that choice reaction time is longer than simple reaction time.

Hick–Hyman Law

The effect on reaction time of increasing the number of stimuli was examined in the early 1950s by Hick (1952) and Hyman (1953). Although they carried out their experiments independently of one another, they came to the same conclusion. They found that as you doubled the number of stimulus–response couplings the reaction time increased. If the reaction time is plotted against the log of the stimulus–response couplings there is a linear increase. This is known as the *Hick–Hyman Law* (Figure 4.4). Generally, reaction time increases by about 150 ms every time the stimulus–response groupings are doubled.

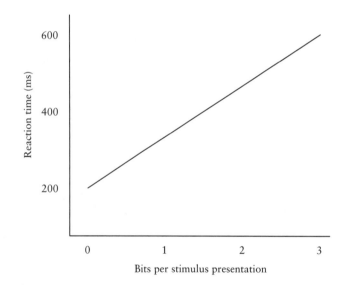

Figure 4.4   Graphical depiction of the Hick–Hyman Law (adapted from Hyman, 1953)

The discerning reader will no doubt have already spotted that, if this is the case, how can we explain the speed at which individuals are able to produce responses in situations where the number of stimuli and possible responses are extremely high? If we take a field hockey goalkeeper facing a penalty flick, there are numerous parts of the goal where the attacker might place the ball. The time it would take to react in such a situation would make it impossible to save a penalty flick. Yet in reality goalkeepers do save penalties. A tennis player facing a 190 km/h (110 mph) serve would have about 480 ms to respond. Glencross and Cibich (1977) stated that reaction time could be shortened, in such situations, by the use of anticipation, which we will examine in detail in the next chapter.

Probability and choice reaction time

One of the ways in which anticipation aids the speeding up of reaction time is to allow the person to predetermine the most likely action that an opponent will take. How this anticipation occurs is covered in the next chapter, but here we will examine the process by which such anticipation shortens reaction time. Unfortunately, research has been limited to situations in which the player can narrow down the number of stimuli to two possibilities. This, of course, is limited in its explanation of how we cope in real-life sporting situations when, even with the use of anticipation, we may have difficulty in narrowing down the possibilities to only two.

Research examining the effect of the probability of the occurrence of a stimulus on the reaction time to that stimulus has generally followed similar protocols. An individual's reaction time, when the stimulus has a 50 per cent chance of being presented, is compared to that when there is a 90 per cent chance. Such research has shown unequivocally that reaction time to the 90 per cent probability stimulus is significantly faster than that to the 50 per cent probability stimulus. Similarly, when there is an 80 per cent probability the reaction time has generally, but not always, been shown to be significantly shorter than that to a 50 per cent chance. Reaction time when probability is decreased to 70 per cent has generally proven to be no faster than that to a 50 per cent probability stimulus.

Two theories have been put forward to explain why reaction time should be shortened when probability is increased. Alain and Proteau (1980) claimed that the person attends to the most likely stimulus at the expense of the less likely one. Dillon, Crassini and Abernethy (1989) argued that the individual stores the responses in a hierarchical order, ready for retrieval. Hence the response to the 90 per cent or 80 per cent probability stimulus is stored ready for recall at the expense of the 10 per cent or 20 per cent stimulus. Whereas, in a 50–50 situation neither is preferred. Dillon, Crassini and Abernethy claimed that the CNS has chosen 70 per cent as a threshold because it calculates that there is no significant advantage in storing the response to that stimulus above that of the 30 per cent chance stimulus. It is, of course, possible that we attend to the most likely stimulus *and* store the responses hierarchically. The research of Alain and Proteau, and Dillon, Crassini and Abernethy suggests that, whatever method is used, it is done so at a sub-conscious level. Their participants were not aware of making a conscious decision as to what to do.

The implications for sport are clear – determine the most likely stimulus and prepare the most likely response. However, much more research is needed. This is particularly so when there will be more than two options. This, of course, is the case in most sports situations.

Psychological refractory period

You may remember that when we discussed the need for selective attention, in Chapter 2, we talked about the limited capacity of the CNS to deal with several things at once. One of the strongest pieces of evidence for this is a phenomenon called the *psychological refractory period*. Research has shown that *when two stimuli are presented close together the reaction time to the second stimulus is slower than the normal reaction time* (Welford, 1968). This is thought to be because the individual cannot process the information from stimulus two until stimulus one has been dealt with. Or at least the person's ability to deal with stimulus two is hampered by having to simultaneously process stimulus one. Figure 4.5 shows a diagrammatic representation of the psychological refractory period.

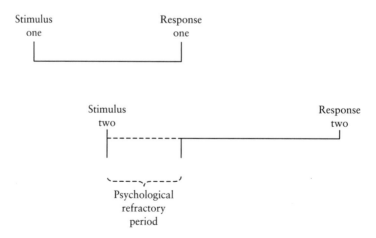

Figure 4.5 Psychological refractory period (adapted from Welford, 1968); reproduced by permission of Thomson Publishing Services from Welford, A.T. 1968 *Fundamentals of Skill*, Methuen, London, UK

The situation is not as simple as Figure 4.5 might suggest. The timing of the presentation of stimulus two is crucial. If stimulus two is presented within 50 ms of stimulus one, the two stimuli can be grouped together and *reacted to as though they were one stimulus*. Research in laboratory tests has shown that practice can reduce the psychological refractory period *but not eliminate it*.

The effect of the psychological refractory period can be seen in many sports. Any example of a feint, dodge or dummy is an example of the use of the psychological refractory period. The feint is stimulus one and the actual movement is stimulus two. If the timing is correct, the defender will be comparatively slow in reacting to the real movement. This is the skill of Rugby players like Jason Robinson, basketball players like Jason King and soccer players such as Ronaldo. Similar feints can be seen in the drop shot in badminton or a dummy punch in boxing. Perhaps the most graphic example of the psychological refractory period in sport is when a goalkeeper is 'wrong footed' by a deflection. The original shot is stimulus one, while the deflection is stimulus two. In such situations the goalkeeper can look as though he/she is 'rooted to the spot'. They have time to abort the response to stimulus one but not to initiate the response to stimulus two.

In many sports, defenders try to overcome the problem of the psychological refractory period by treating the two stimuli as one, even if they occur more than 50 ms apart. If a player knows that an opponent uses a particular dummy or feint, he/she will use stimulus one as a warning that stimulus two will appear. As such, they can actually produce a faster than normal reaction to stimulus two. However, if the opponent is playing a 'double bluff', reaction time to stimulus one will be considerably slower than normal reaction time.

Arousal and reaction time

Although the effect of arousal on reaction time is one of the most researched areas of motor performance, it is difficult to make a definitive statement about it. Despite this, in most textbooks you will see it stated that arousal affects reaction time in line with the Yerkes–Dodson Law. According to Yerkes and Dodson (1908), moderate intensity arousal produces the fastest reaction times, while high and low levels elicit slow reaction times. In Chapter 10, we examine the effect of arousal on all forms of performance in some detail. As a result we will simply outline the basics of the theory here.

Easterbrook's (1959) cue utilization theory explains how the Yerkes–Dodson Law works by stating that at low levels of arousal the person's focus is susceptible to distraction from non-relevant stimuli, so the reaction time is comparatively long. At moderate levels, the attention has narrowed onto task relevant cues only, therefore the reaction time is short. While at high levels, there is too much narrowing and relevant cues are missed, resulting in long reaction times. As we will see in Chapter 10, this claim has been challenged by more recent theories. More importantly, research findings do not fully support the claims of either Yerkes and Dodson or Easterbrook. It is difficult, however, to compare research, as the cause of the arousal and type of response required differ greatly from one experiment to another. Suffice it to say, at this stage, that arousal can affect reaction time.

Anecdotal evidence exists for a reaction time–arousal interaction. Watch a substitute enter a game. Often the game appears to 'go on around them' until they get warmed-up. We also need only think about our reactions when we wake up in the morning compared with later in the day or our reactions when we are tired. As we will see in Chapter 10, our anecdotal evidence may, however, not be as good as we might think.

Stimulus and response factors

Intra-individual differences in reaction time are often the result of altering the nature of the stimulus and/or response or the stimulus–response interaction effect. The first two factors that we will examine have already been looked at when we considered Signal Detection Theory in Chapter 2. The *intensity of the stimulus or signal* affects reaction time. We react faster to the more intense signals. Signal Detection Theory would suggest that this is because *d*-prime is greater. It could, however, simply be because we may be programmed to attend to stimuli that may be threatening and we assume intense signals to be such.

The second factor that we have already examined is *stimulus familiarity*. There appears to be little doubt that we react faster to stimuli with which we are familiar compared with unfamiliar stimuli. This has major implications for practice. If we react faster to familiar stimuli then we should practice using these stimuli. It is for this reason that boxers will spar against someone using a similar style to that which their next opponent uses. Similarly, in the martial arts and military situations realistic stimuli are used in practice.

Another major factor affecting the stimulus–reaction time interaction is the *sensory modality* of the stimulus. As reaction time to visual stimuli is what we are most used to, one might expect it to be the shortest. In fact, it is not. Reaction time to auditory stimuli is shorter. The proximity of the auditory nerves to the CNS allows information to be passed very quickly to the sensory cortex. Although the eyes are also very near to the CNS, the visual information entering is in the form of light waves and has to be transduced into electrical nerve impulses before stimulating the retinal nerves. As a result visual reaction time is greater that auditory. Mean simple visual reaction time is between 170 and 200 ms in normal adults, while auditory reaction time is around the 100 ms mark. The difference between visual and auditory reaction time is, however, dependent on other factors. The basic difference explained above does not take into account factors such as signal intensity and stimulus familiarity. It is very difficult, if not impossible, to ensure that two stimuli, activating two different senses, are of the same intensity. How can you compare the intensity of a sound to the intensity of a visual stimulus?

The difference between speed to visual and auditory stimuli compared to that to tactile stimuli is dependent on where the tactile stimulus is applied. A tactile stimulus applied to the face may well produce a very fast reaction compared to one applied to the foot, simply due to the distance from the CNS. However, reaction time to the stimulus to the foot may be very fast if it is dealt with by the spinal chord rather than the CNS. Information Processing theorists have tended to describe such reactions as being part of the *reflex arc* and, as such, not a true reaction. This is a very debatable point and is dealt with in some detail in Chapter 7, when we examine the way in which movement is controlled.

While the nature of the sensory mode will affect reaction time so will the length of the *foreperiod*. The foreperiod is the time between the presentation of a warning signal and the onset of the stimulus. Foreperiods can be too short, giving the person little time to prepare a response. Or they can be too long. The individual is not able to maintain attention and/or physical readiness. We often see this in sprint races when competitors have to stand up in order to stop themselves false starting. There is considerable disagreement as to the actual foreperiod that will elicit optimal reaction time. It would appear that it is dependent on the nature of the response required. More complex responses need more time to be prepared. The most dramatic effect on foreperiods, however, can be seen from research into constant versus random foreperiods. Constant foreperiods lead to short, in fact very short, reaction times. The individual uses the warning to aid anticipation of when the stimulus is to be presented. Quesada and Schmidt (1970) demonstrated mean reaction times of as little as 22 ms in such circumstances.

With regard to the ways in which responses affect reaction time there are two major factors. The first is the number of responses for which we need to prepare. As we have seen, choice reaction time is greater than simple reaction time where there is only one possible response. This is because, in a choice reaction-time situation, the individual must prepare a number of responses before determining which is the most appropriate. In a simple reaction-time situation, the decision and efferent organization are pre-planned, and therefore the individual only needs to perceive the stimulus in order to act.

In some sports having a wide range of techniques available in any given situation can have a detrimental effect on speed of reaction. The performer who is limited technically can only prepare one or two possible responses, while the more gifted performer will prepare more. This, in itself, takes more time but the situation is exacerbated by the fact that the performer must then choose between the possible options as well.

The second major factor, with regard to the response, is the *response complexity*. The more complex the response the longer the preparation. The greater the neuropsychological demands the longer the reaction time. This can, however, be offset to a large extent if performing the motor act becomes automatic. Watching experienced sprinters we see that they can respond very quickly to the gun, despite the fact that the movement is quite complex. Cricket and baseball batters are probably a better example because their responses require not only complex movements but also timing.

Although the above are all large factors affecting reaction time, it is probably the stimulus–response interaction that has the largest affect. As stated above, familiarity with the stimulus and automaticity of response both affect reaction time. When we place them together, i.e., the person has to react to a familiar stimulus using a response which they can do automatically, reaction time can be very short indeed.

A factor similar to this is *response compatibility*. Research in laboratories has shown that if the required response is in the same direction as the stimulus, reaction time is faster than if the response is in a different direction. For example, in some experiments the person has to point a lever towards the stimulus when it is presented, while in others they have to move a different lever or move the same lever but in the opposite direction to the stimulus. Response compatibility in real-life situations is less obvious. In some situations it will be compatible to move towards a stimulus, e.g., a ball to be caught, but in others it will be compatible to move away from the object, e.g., a punch. Research has shown that practice can eliminate a non-compatibility effect, therefore performers going into situations for which the response is non-compatible will need plenty of time to practice. An example of such a response would be getting into the line of flight of a fast ball coming at you in cricket. It is not a normal reaction yet it is the one that will allow the best chance of hitting the ball.

As we have seen above, when a response becomes automatic it takes less time to process. It also allows the individual to focus on the stimulus when preparing a response. Research has shown that focusing on the stimulus rather the response aids reaction time. This is called using the *sensory set*. Linford Christie alluded to this when he said that the hurdler Colin Jackson had told him to go on the 'b' of the 'bang'. In other words, concentrate on the sound of the gun, not the motor act. Attending to the motor action is called using the *motor set*. Nevertheless, we often see coaches telling their runners to concentrate on the movement rather than the gun. Sprinters should ensure that the movement is automatic, then concentrate on starting quickly.

Reaction-time research findings as evidence for Information Processing Theory

To the Information Processing theorists, the fact that research unequivocally demonstrates that it takes time to act is proof that the CNS is the key factor in performance. This claim is, they say, strengthened by the fact that it is the manipulation of factors such as the number of stimuli to be processed and the familiarity of the stimuli that result in an increase in reaction time. According to Information Processing theorists, altering the nature of the stimuli changes the load placed on working memory. Therefore, if reaction time is increased when the number of stimuli are increased, it is because the demands on working memory become greater. Similarly, they argue that increases in reaction time, when the response to be made is complex or has high neuropsychological demands, shows that efferent organization is being affected. This is also shown when a response becomes automatic and reaction time decreases because it requires less processing time. This, the Information Processing theorists say, is because automaticity means that efferent organization takes less space in the information-processing channel.

Without any fear of contradiction, we can say that there is a limitation on how quickly we can perform. When the number and nature of the stimuli and responses are altered reaction time is affected. To the Information Processing theorists, this is mainly due to the way in which these changes affect opto-motor integration time. The problem appears to be the load that the stimuli and responses place on the information-processing channel.

Key points

- Response time is the time from the introduction of a stimulus until the completion of a response:

- ○ response time consists of reaction time plus movement time.

- Reaction time is the time from the sudden onset of a stimulus until the beginning of an overt response.

- Reaction time can be divided into:

  - ○ reception time (time taken for information to be transmitted from the senses to the sensory cortex),

  - ○ opto-motor integration time (time for the CNS to decide what to do and to organize the movement),

  - ○ motor outflow time (time for the efferent information to be transmitted to the limbs),

  - ○ motor time (time taken for the muscles to be activated by the efferent nerves).

- Reaction time can be:
  - ○ simple (one stimulus and one response),
  - ○ choice (several stimuli and several responses).

- Choice reaction time is longer than simple reaction time:

  - ○ Hick–Hyman Law states that as the number of possible stimulus–response couplings are increased so reaction time increases,

  - ○ the increase in reaction time is linear.

- If a stimulus is likely to occur at above 70 per cent of the time, reaction time to that stimulus will be shorter than reaction time when there is a 50 per cent chance of the stimulus being presented.

- When two stimuli are presented close together, reaction time to the second stimulus is longer than normal reaction time – this is due to the psychological refractory period:

- the second stimulus cannot be processed until the beginning of movement time for the first stimulus,

- if the two stimuli are presented within 50 ms of one another, they can be treated as one stimulus,

- practice can limit the effect of the psychological refractory period but not eliminate it.

- Arousal is thought to affect reaction time in an inverted-U fashion:

  - high and low arousal result in long reaction times,

  - moderate arousal causes short reaction times.

- The stimulus can result in short reaction times if:

  - it is intense in comparison with the background noise,

  - it is familiar.

- Auditory reaction time is shorter than visual and tactile.

- Foreperiods can affect reaction time:

  - constant foreperiods lead to very short reaction times due to anticipation,

  - very short foreperiods result in long reaction times, as the person does not have time to prepare the response,

  - long foreperiods result in long reaction times because the individual is not able to maintain physical readiness long enough,

  - foreperiods of moderate length produce short reaction times.

- The nature of the response can affect reaction time:

  - complex responses require a lot of processing, therefore reaction times are long,

○ the greater the number of possible responses, the longer the reaction time,

○ compatible responses (responses in the same direction as the stimulus) produce shorter reaction times than non-compatible responses.

• The individual's psychological set (what they are focusing on prior to responding) can affect reaction time:

○ sensory set (focusing on the stimulus) leads to a shorter reaction time than

○ motor set (focusing on the response).

Test your knowledge

(Answers in Appendix 3.)

Part one

Complete the following sentences using the phrases below.

1. Response time consists of _____.

2. Reaction time is the time that elapses from the sudden onset of a stimulus to _____.

3. Reaction time consists of _____.

4. Simple reaction time is when there is only _____.

5. 170 to 200 ms represents the _____.

6. According to the Hick–Hyman Law, as the number of stimuli–response combinations is increased, reaction time _____.

7. If a stimulus has a 90 per cent probability of being presented, it will demonstrate a reaction time that is shorter than if _____.

8. Dillon, Crassini and Abernethy (1989) claimed that a stimulus with a 90 per cent probability of presentation would be reacted to quickly because we _____.

9. Reaction times, when the probability of a stimulus being presented is 70 per cent and when it is 50 per cent, show _____.

10. The psychological refractory period shows that when two stimuli are presented close together reaction time to the second stimulus will be _____.

11. Practice can reduce the psychological refractory period but _____.

12. If two stimuli are presented within 50 ms of one another they can _____.

13. According to Yerkes and Dodson (1908), a moderate level of arousal will induce a reaction time that is shorter than when arousal level is _____.

14. A shorter than normal reaction time will be shown when the stimulus stands out against _____.

15. Visual reaction time is longer than _____.

16. If a foreperiod is too short, the person does not have _____.

17. Complex responses require longer foreperiods because _____.

one stimulus and one response
range of mean simple reaction times
reaction time and movement time
store responses in a hierarchical order
longer than normal
increases linearly

the response takes longer to prepare   the background
cannot eliminate it   low or high
auditory   pre-motor and motor time
the beginning of an overt response   time to prepare the response
no significant difference   it has a 50 per cent chance
treated as one

Part two

Which of the following statements are true (T) and which are false (F)?

1. Movement time is the time from the beginning of an overt
    response to the completion of an action.   T   F

2. A person can have a short reaction time but a long movement
    time.   T   F

3. Reception time and motor outflow time are controlled by
    the CNS.   T   F

4. In choice reaction-time situations, opto-motor integration
    time is responsible for inter- and intra-individual differences.   T   F

5. Motor time differs greatly from one person to another.   T   F

6. The efficiency of working memory will affect choice reaction
    time.   T   F

7. Research into probability and reaction time suggests that the
    strategy used to shorten reaction time is consciously chosen. T   F

8. Alain and Proteau (1980) stated that, when one stimulus is
    90 per cent certain of being presented, we focus on that
    stimulus at the expense of other stimuli.   T   F

9. According to Easterbrook (1953), when arousal is high we
    focus on relevant and irrelevant information.   T   F

10. According to Easterbrook (1953), when arousal is low we
    focus on relevant and irrelevant information.   T   F

11. Practice using a particular stimulus cannot improve reaction
    time to that stimulus.   T   F

12.	Speed of reaction to a tactile stimulus is the same no matter which part of the body is stimulated.	T	F
13.	Visual reaction time is longer than auditory because light waves need to be transduced into electrical nerve impulses before the information can be passed to the CNS.	T	F
14.	There is no such thing as a reflex arc.	T	F
15.	In a reaction time task, if the foreperiod is too long the individual cannot hold the ready position.	T	F
16.	Randomizing foreperiods leads to shorter reaction times than using constant foreperiods.	T	F
17.	Practising a response, so that it becomes automatic, helps reduce reaction time.	T	F
18.	Practice cannot reduce the effect of response compatibility on reaction time.	T	F
19.	Using the sensory set means focusing on the response rather than the stimulus.	T	F
20.	Information Processing theorists claim that as choice reaction time is longer than simple reaction time, action must be controlled by the CNS.	T	F

Additional reading

Greene J and Hicks C (1991) *Basic cognitive processes*. Open University Press, Milton Keynes, UK

Welford AT (Ed) (1973) *Reaction time*. Academic Press, London, UK

5 Anticipation

Learning Objectives

By the end of this chapter, you should be able to

- understand what is meant by interceptive actions
- understand how Information Processing Theory explains interceptive actions, with reference to
    - ◊ receptor anticipation
    - ◊ effector anticipation
    - ◊ role of working memory
- understand how Action Systems Theory explains interceptive actions, with reference to
    - ◊ tau(τ)
- understand the nature and role of perceptual anticipation in skilled performance
- understand how Information Processing Theory explains perceptual information, with reference to
    - ◊ working memory
- understand how Action Systems Theory explains perceptual anticipation with reference to
    - ◊ attunement to affordances
- understand the difficulties of carrying out research into anticipation
- understand the main research findings into anticipation

Acquisition and Performance of Sports Skills   T. McMorris
© 2004 John Wiley & Sons, Ltd   ISBNs: 0-470-84994-0 (HB); 0-470-84995-9 (PB)

Introduction

In the last two chapters, we have alluded to how anticipation helps us to determine what is going to happen before it actually does happen. Thus, we are able to make decisions and respond very quickly. This type of anticipation is called *perceptual anticipation* and is what the lay person is likely to think of when talking about anticipation. Anticipation, however, also explains how we are able to undertake *interceptive actions*. Interceptive actions are skills such as catching, hitting or kicking a moving object. This may require very fast reactions, such as receiving a fast serve in tennis or hitting a baseball pitched at 180 km/h (100 mph). However, it also applies when the object is moving slowly. We will discuss perceptual anticipation later in this chapter but in the first section we examine anticipation for interceptive actions.

Interceptive actions are the bases of many sports. Hitting a tennis ball, kicking a soccer ball or catching a netball are all examples of interceptive actions. Interceptive actions may also include stopping an opponent's movement as in Rugby or American Football. Even punching someone in boxing is an interceptive action. We should also consider avoiding interception as being a form of 'interceptive action', albeit a negative interceptive action. Avoiding a punch in boxing is a good example of such a skill.

Interceptive actions

Information Processing Theory and interceptive actions

Poulton (1957) called the making of interceptive actions *coincidence anticipation*. Sometimes the term *coincidence timing* is used. Coincidence anticipation is, according to Poulton, the combination of two different forms of anticipation, effector anticipation and receptor anticipation. *Effector anticipation* refers to the individual's ability to determine how long it will take him/her to move their limbs. While *receptor anticipation* is the ability to decide how long it will take an external event to happen. So, for example, in catching a ball (the interceptive action) the person needs to anticipate how long it will take the ball to come into range so that the catch can be made (receptor anticipation) and how long it will take them to get their hands into position (effector anticipation). The more discerning among you will realize that simply getting your hands into position will not necessarily mean that the catch will be made successfully. The individual also needs to anticipate how quickly they will need to 'give' when the ball and hands make contact.

The example of catching the ball shows that coincidence anticipation can require a great deal of anticipatory skill. Hitting a forehand drive in tennis also requires a high level of anticipatory skill, especially if the individual is to hit the ball hard. Following Newton's Laws of Motion, we know that action and reaction are equal and opposite. Therefore, if the timing of the hand and arm movements (effector anticipation) are such that they meet the ball at a point level with the player's body, a great deal of power will be demonstrated. The person does not need to be very strong to achieve this and the faster the ball comes the better, if the timing is correct. The cricketer Brian Lara is a good example of someone whose timing allows him to hit the ball much harder than would be expected from a 1.7 m (5 foot 6 inch) tall man of average build. Cricketers like Lara are also able to make shots that require very minimal bat–ball contact in order to deflect the ball from its original path, e.g., playing a leg glance. McLeod and Jenkins (1991) showed that, in order to play a leg glance stroke, the cricketer has only a 4 ms error margin. The beginner often reacts too slowly but the expert can repeatedly hit balls moving at 140–190 km/h (80–90 mph). Also, soccer and hockey players controlling the ball need to time their interception to a very high degree of accuracy.

According to the Information Processing theorists, when we make an interceptive action we judge the speed and trajectory (line of flight) of the object, calculate how long it will take for the object to reach a position in which we can make an interception and, in addition, determine how long it will take our limbs to get into position to make the interception. The ability to do this can be best explained by examining the whole of the Information Processing model (see Figure 1.4). It should be of no surprise to you, by now, that the Information Processing theorists see the ability to carry out these skills as relying very heavily on past experience stored in the LTM. Experience of having to make interceptive actions, or even just observing the speed and trajectory of moving objects, builds up a LTM store that aids the perceptual, decision-making and efferent organization necessary to make a successful interception.

So far we have only considered the decision-making aspect of interceptive actions in respect to timing. That is not the only role of decision making during interception. The person needs to decide not only *when* to make the interception but also *how* to make it. In other words, which technique needs to be used in order to make the most successful interceptive action. Examining catching can help us to understand this. Whether we catch the ball with our fingers pointing upwards or downwards and whether we use one or two hands affects our efficiency. The knowledge of which technique is best, in any given situation, is dependent on past experience.

To support this argument, the Information Processing theorists point to developmental factors in catching a ball. Developmental psychologists have shown that young children (3 years old) try to use the same technique to catch a ball no matter what the size of the ball or if the trajectory is high or low. As they get older (5 years old) and more experienced they will change the technique to be used depending on the ball trajectory and position. Similarly, one of the key factors in the child developing the skill of catching is the understanding of when and how far to 'give' when the hands make contact with the ball. This does not happen until the child has considerable experience of trying to catch a ball. Differences in the rate at which children show these developments are due to the amount and nature of the child's experiences.

Watching the object to be intercepted

It is common to hear cricket coaches tell their players to 'watch the ball onto the bat'. Tennis, table tennis and badminton coaches give similar instructions. Our ability to do this has been questioned for some time. Hubbard and Seng (1954) watched film of baseball batters hitting fast pitches. They observed that the batters stopped trying to follow the ball with their eyes, when the ball was between 2.7 and 1.7 m (9 and 5.5 feet) from the point of contact. They argued that the time it took for the ball to travel this short distance meant that any alteration in movement was impossible due to the limitations of reaction time.

However, more recent research by Bootsma and Van Wieringen (1990), examining table tennis players and using more sophisticated equipment, showed that players were able to make *some* adjustments to their bat swing very late in flight. These alterations were small and merely consisted of a refinement of the chosen movement. Similarly, research (Davids and Stratford, 1989) has shown that occluding the vision of the hand in catching experiments inhibits performance. However, experience can compensate to a limited extent. It would appear that watching the object all the way to the point of interception is of some, albeit limited, use.

Action Systems Theory and interceptive actions

To the ecological psychologists, particularly those taking an Action Systems stance, all the information we need in order to make an interceptive action is present in the environment. Visual information provides all of the perceptual information necessary to intercept an object. As we saw in Chapter 2, light waves from the person's eyes to the object to be intercepted and back again provide information about the line and speed of flight. According to David Lee (e.g., Lee and Young, 1985), this information is all we need in order to know when the object will make contact with us. Lee argued that the rate at which the size of the image of the object on the retina increased allowed us to know the *time to contact*. Lee called this time to contact by the Greek letter *tau* (τ) and developed a mathematical formula to explain how it worked. It is not in the scope of an introductory text, such as this, to examine the formula but suffice it to say that the key factor is the rate of change of the retinal image, rather than actual size of the object or the distance from which it comes, that allows us to determine τ. Figures 2.3(a) to (c) provide a good example of the change in the size of the image, however they cannot demonstrate the rate of change as there is no motion. We have all, however, experienced situations when watching television and an object appears to be coming towards us and we move to avoid contact, even though we know it cannot come out of the television set.

Although τ explains receptor anticipation, it does not explain effector anticipation. Action Systems Theory, however, provides a simple explanation. When contact is imminent, the object provides an affordance to make or avoid contact. For example, fielders in cricket and baseball are constantly searching for the opportunity, or affordance, to catch the ball. τ tells them when this is possible and the necessary movement is taken care of automatically. This is an example of perception–action coupling. The individual does not need recourse to memory in order to determine the timing and nature of the hand movements necessary to catch the ball.

Ironically, although Lee is an ecological psychologist his τ hypothesis has been criticized on the grounds that it lacks ecological validity. The determination of τ is based on the assumption that the speed of the approaching object is constant. This, of course, is not the case in most sporting situations. A ball does not travel at a constant speed after being hit or kicked towards you. Lee accepted this criticism and claimed that the individual automatically takes this into account and, in such situations, determines what he calls *tau dot* ($\dot{\tau}$). Lee provides a mathematical model for this explanation. This model is generally accepted by ecological psychologists. Furthermore, recent research by Lenoir *et al.* (1999) has examined the way in which catchers move in order to take in the most pertinent information to allow them to make a catch. Results have not been unequivocal but it can be said that it appears that catchers try to get their head into positions that allow them to optimally perceive the rate of change of the retinal image. This can easily be seen when we watch cricketers and baseball players manoeuvering to take a high catch.

Perceptual anticipation

Perceptual anticipation is the *ability of the performer to predict upcoming events based on partial information*. The partial information will normally be in the form of cues unfolding in the display. Perceptual anticipation plays a major role in helping us to respond in situations that require a decision to be made in shorter than one reaction time. It is these kinds of situations, which have attracted the most attention, but it should be remembered that perceptual anticipation also plays a major role in the way we make decisions when not under time pressure.

Information Processing Theory and perceptual anticipation

The kinds of anticipation that make up perceptual anticipation are spatial, temporal and event. *Spatial* anticipation refers to *where* an individual thinks an action will occur. *Temporal* anticipation, of course, refers to the timing of an action or *when* something will occur, while *event* anticipation is the determination of *what* will happen. Perceptual anticipation can include one or all of these factors, depending on the situation. In most of the situations we will be examining in this section all three are important but particularly event anticipation.

Unless you have skipped the last four chapters, it will be of no surprise to find that the Information Processing Theory explanation of perceptual anticipation places great emphasis on past experience held in the LTM. The key issues are selective attention and pattern recognition. Selective attention allows the person to know which areas of the display to search for relevant cues. While pattern recognition is the ability to recognize, from only partial information, what is about to happen. The Information Processing theorists point to the large amount of research that has examined expert–novice differences to support their claims that experience is the vital factor affecting perceptual anticipation. Experts invariably outperform novices in sports-specific perceptual anticipation tasks. Indeed, some research has shown that experts do better than intermediate-level performers, although this is not unequivocal.

Many Information Processing theorists believe that although perceptual anticipation is dependent on memory, it can be a *conscious* or *non-conscious* activity. In Chapter 1, we discussed the possibility of perception taking place in a non-conscious way and we will examine non-conscious or implicit learning in Chapter 8. The argument that perceptual anticipation may be non-conscious comes about because often we cannot articulate how we 'knew' that something was going to happen – we just 'knew'.

Ecological psychology and perceptual anticipation

As perceptual anticipation is primarily a CNS function, ecological psychologists have little to say about it. To them perceptual anticipation depends on the recognition of events, which will lead to certain affordances. It is not a product of memory. All of the information required is present in the environment. To the ecological psychologist, a tennis player anticipating whether an opponent will return the ball down the line or across court can do so from the *biomechanical* information that the opponent provides. The position of the body parts and the racket provide all the necessary information. If you look at Figure 5.1, you can see that it is not possible for the player to play a cross-court shot, given his body position. Ecological psychologists would support the claim that perceptual anticipation takes place subconsciously. It is a form of attunement to affordances.

Research paradigms in perceptual anticipation

The first people to research perceptual anticipation were Jones and Miles (1978). They examined the ability of amateur tennis players and experienced tennis coaches to anticipate where serves would land. The research paradigm used by Jones and Miles was what we call a *temporal occlusion* paradigm. It has been used by many researchers since. Jones and Miles showed their participants film clips of a player serving. They froze the action at certain chosen times: two frames before racket–ball contact, at contact and two frames after contact. The participants were given a scaled map of a tennis court and had to mark down, on the map, where they thought the ball would land. Jones and Miles measured the distance from where the participant thought the ball would land to where it had actually landed. The amount of error is called *radial error*. The differences in radial error between amateurs and coaches and between the occlusion points were compared. Later researchers have measured

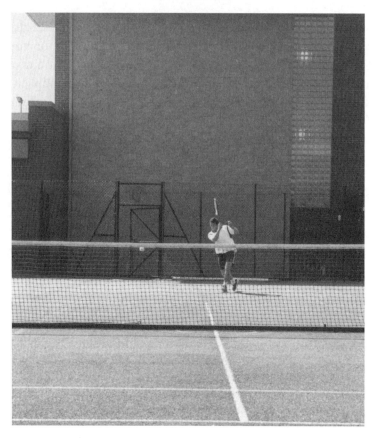

Figure 5.1 Tennis player playing a forehand drive down the line (note that his body position shows that it is impossible for him to play cross court)

lateral and depth error, as well as radial error. Figure 5.2 shows how to calculate these.

There is no doubt that this research design has provided us with some very interesting data. It is, of course, not without its problems. Using a scaled map to show where you think the ball would bounce is difficult. Try it for yourself. Get someone to place objects on a table and measure the distances from the edges of the table, so that they know exactly where the object was placed. Then get them to draw two scaled maps of the table, one on transparent acetate paper. On the acetate paper get them to mark exactly where the objects are. Using the other map try to mark where the objects were, yourself. Place the transparent acetate on top of your paper and measure the radial error. You will see that it is not easy to be accurate *even when you can see the objects in a static display*. In order to overcome this, my colleague Tim Holder (1998), carrying out research on anticipation in table tennis, had the particpants make a mark on a full-size

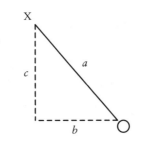

○ Where ball actually landed
X Participant's estimation of where ball landed

a, radial error
b, line or width error
c, length or depth error

Figure 5.2 How to calculate radial, lateral (width) and depth error

table tennis table rather than a scaled-down map. This would appear to be more realistic. However, when Tim compared using a real table with using a scaled map, he found no significant difference.

To the ecological psychologists, using marks on a map or an actual playing area is pointless because it separates perception from action. Indeed, many Information Processing theorists are unhappy with this method of determining anticipation because it is measuring declarative rather than procedural knowledge. The situation is exacerbated by the fact that, using the paradigm of Jones and Miles, participants are sat watching a film or video whereas in real-life situations they would be standing ready for action and have to make a physical response. Clatworthy, Holder and Graydon (1991), testing anticipation of hockey goalkeepers facing penalty flicks, had the goalkeepers stand in front of a back screen projector facing a full-size film of a player taking penalty flicks. The goalkeepers were dressed in full kit and had to respond by simulating 'making a save', i.e., they had to dive or move their stick to the position that they would have done if making a real save. Where they actually moved and where the ball really went were compared. While this appears more realistic, it is not very easy to do and requires a great deal of familiarization by the participants. Moreover, Holder found that there were no significant differences between using this method and marking positions on a map of the actual playing area.

The most prolific researcher into perceptual anticipation is the Australian Bruce Abernethy. Abernethy (1992) began by using temporal occlusion paradigms and examined many sports. While his temporal occlusion research produced valuable information, he was not satisfied with simply ascertaining whether experts could use pre-ball release or pre-bat(racket)–ball contact cues to anticipate. He wanted to know what cues were providing the most valuable information. In order to do this he developed the *spatial occlusion* paradigm. In this he 'blacked out' players' body parts or the racket when examining badminton (Abernethy and Russell, 1987). If anticipation decreased when a particular part was blacked out that part must be providing a great deal of useful information to the anticipator. The major problem facing Abernethy, however, was the technology of the time. I have placed 'blacked out' in inverted commas because, in fact, the part was merely distorted, as we see on television when someone's face is blocked to avoid identity. Nevertheless, it was a very innovative method and provided much very useful research. With modern advances in computers, it is now possible to make something disappear from view totally.

Spatial occlusion paradigms require the researcher to predetermine the parts of the display that they think will provide valuable information to the anticipator. With the aid of experienced and qualified coaches, this would appear to be a not too difficult task. However, to many researchers this is too great an assumption. They, therefore, wished to know exactly what performers were looking at when anticipating. The development of *eye-mark recorders* made this possible. Eye-mark recorders show where the person is focusing his/her gaze. They have been used in research examining which body and racket parts are focused on by tennis players (Goulet, Bard and Fleury, 1989) and what parts of the player and stick ice hockey goaltenders examined when facing a slap shot (Salmela and Fiorito, 1979). They have also been used to examine areas of the display that basketball (Allard, Graham and Paarsalu, 1980), volleyball (Allard and Starkes, 1980) and soccer (Williams and Davids, 1998) players examine when anticipating what action opponents will take. Eye-mark recorders have been used when participants were looking at videos of action and also in real-life situations. The latter has a major advantage over the former in that the anticipator sees everything in three dimensions rather than the two dimensions perceived in a video. However, in real-life situations it is not possible for the researcher to control the movements of the opponents, therefore valuable information may be missed. I would imagine that virtual reality would provide the vehicle for the next paradigm to be developed in perceptual anticipation research.

Research findings

Most research into perceptual anticipation has examined expert–novice differences. Research examining anticipation of where a ball would land, using temporal occlusion paradigms, has unequivocally shown experts to be better than novices, regardless of the types of measures that were used – marking a position on a map, marking a position on the actual target or using a real movement. This is hardly unexpected. Indeed, if it were not the case it would be more interesting. In itself, it says very little. Of more interest is the research showing that novices *can learn* to use perceptual anticipation.

Research examining expert–intermediate-level differences has shown that experts anticipate better; however, results have not been unequivocal. At first this may appear to be surprising but when we consider the nature of skill perhaps it is not so. In a skill in which perceptual anticipation is important, it is very unlikely that one can reach expert status without demonstrating good anticipation. In skills where it is less important other abilities may make up for comparative weaknesses. For example, an American Football lineman does not need very much perceptual anticipatory skill because his responses are predetermined by the coach. He does, however, have to be big, very big. On the other hand, a defensive back requires good perceptual anticipation. It should, also, be remembered that an intermediate-level player may have very good anticipatory skills but be lacking in other abilities which are necessary to reach expert level. For example, a stand-off in Rugby, who has good perceptual anticipation but is not a very fast runner, may perform well at intermediate level but is not going to reach top-class level. This is a good example of the ability–skill interaction and the changing task factor covered in Chapter 1.

Research using spatial occlusion designs has also focused on expert–novice differences. As we saw with the research of Fran Allard and her colleagues, in Chapter 2, there are significant differences in what the two groups look at. The differences are not only in the order of the search but also in the time spent examining each cue. Experts examine areas of the display that are generally considered, by coaches, to provide a great deal of information. Moreover, they spend more time than novices focusing on these areas. Research into visual search in team games strongly supports this. However, research into what players look at, when competing against an individual, have provided some surprising results.

In racket games, the old adage 'keep your eye on the ball' does not appear to be used by experts. Several researchers have shown that racket games players focus on the arm carrying the racket. However, one should be very careful in drawing any conclusions based on this research because it was undertaken in the laboratory, with the participant sitting to watch a video of their opponent. Research carried out in more ecologically valid situations suggests this may not be the case. Ripoll and Latiri (1997) showed that, in matchplay, table tennis players watch bat–ball contact more than anything else. In fast ball games, it appears to me that you cannot totally take your eye off the ball if you are going to successfully intercept it. However, this does not mean that you do not perceive the ball peripherally. In a fascinating experiment, Mark Williams and Keith Davids (1998) examined what semi-professional soccer players focus on when defending in a one versus one situation. They found that the players focused mainly on an area around their opponent's hips. At first this sounds crazy. Surely, they would watch the ball or their opponent's feet. However, by focusing on the hip area the player can take in information from the ball and feet but can, also, take in information from the upper body, which may be useful.

Conclusion

We use anticipation to allow us to make interceptive actions. To the Information Processing theorists, we develop this ability by building up a LTM store concerning the speed and trajectory of the objects that need to be intercepted and the speed of our own movements. To the ecological psychologists, this information is present in the environment and is not affected by memory.

We also use anticipation to help us to make fast responses. Again to the Information Processing theorists, this ability is memory driven while, to the ecological psychologists, successful performance is due to an interaction with the environment and all necessary information is detected by searching the display. Both Information Processing theorists and ecological psychologists accept that perceptual anticipation aids visual search and, hence, selective attention. Moreover, both schools believe that experience in the specific environment, in which the anticipation is to be made, is necessary for perceptual anticipation ability to develop.

The ecological psychologists have been critical of the laboratory-based research used by many Information Processing theorists. However, comparison of findings between methods of varying ecological validity tend to show the same results. Nevertheless, the lack of research comparing experts to intermediates leaves one uneasy about the strength of the claims of many researchers. The separation of perception and action is particularly disturbing. More research in ecologically valid situations is required.

Key points

Information Processing Theory and interceptive actions

- Coincidence anticipation (making an interceptive action) can be divided into:

      o   receptor anticipation (anticipation of the time taken for the object to reach you),

      o   effector anticipation (the time it takes you to make the interception).

- Receptor anticipation is dependent on working memory.

Action Systems Theory and interceptive actions

- Perceiving the object to be intercepted and making the interception cannot be separated (perception–action coupling).

- They are dependent on tau (τ, 'calculation' of time to contact):

      o   the rate of change of the size of the image of the object on the retina tells us when contact is imminent,

      o   we respond automatically.

- We are able to allow for the fact that the object does not accelerate in a uniform manner by the 'calculation' of tau dot ($\dot{\tau}$).

Watching the ball and interceptive actions

- The last part of flight may be of little use when making an interception:

      o   at best only minor changes can be made.

Information Processing Theory and perceptual anticipation

- Perceptual anticipation is the ability of the performer to predict upcoming events based on partial information.

- Perceptual anticipation predicts where, when and how something might happen.

- Perceptual anticipation is dependent on:

- selective attention,
- pattern recognition,
- working memory.

Ecological psychology and perceptual anticipation

- All of the necessary information is present in the display:

    - biomechanical information tells us about the movement of objects and people.

Research paradigms in perceptual anticipation

- Presentation of videos and film of performance.

- Occlusion paradigms:

    - temporal (e.g., in cricket, the action is stopped at chosen times, normally pre-, at and post-ball release by the bowler),

    - spatial occlusion (e.g., in tennis, parts of a server's body are occluded as he/she serves).

- The person must mark down, on a map of the pitch or court, where they think the object (normally a ball) will land.

- Performance is measured by the amount of error, it can be:

    - radial error (distance in a straight line from the actual landing place),

    - lateral error (distance from the anticipated landing position to a line running vertically from the actual landing place),

    - depth error (distance from the anticipated landing position to a line running horizontally from the actual landing place).

- Visual search paradigms:

- the person's pattern of visual search is determined using eye-mark recorders,

- where the person looked, the length of time spent looking at a particular piece of information and the order of search are all measured.

Research results

- Experts are better than novices:
  - experts are generally, but not always, better than intermediate performers,
  - experts use different search patterns to novices,
  - experts focus longer on areas of relevance.

Test your knowledge

(Answers in Appendix 3.)

Part one

Choose which of the phrases, (a), (b), (c) or (d), best completes the statement or answers the question. There is only *one* correct answer for each problem.

1. Effector anticipation refers to:
   (a) the judgement of the time it takes for external events to happen,
   (b) the judgement of the time it takes for the person to move his/her limbs,
   (c) the timing of an interceptive action,
   (d) the anticipation of where the object is going.

2. Receptor anticipation refers to:
   (a) the judgement of the time it takes for external events to happen,
   (b) the judgement of the time it takes for the person to move his/her limbs,

    (c) the timing of an interceptive action,

    (d) the anticipation of where the object is going.

3. Coincidence anticipation refers to:

    (a) the judgement of the time it takes for external events to happen,

    (b) the judgement of the time it takes for the person to move his/her limbs,

    (c) the timing of an interceptive action,

    (d) the actual time it takes for an external event to happen.

4. According to Information Processing theorists, the ability to judge the speed and trajectory of an object is due to:

    (a) short-term memory,

    (b) long-term memory,

    (c) working memory,

    (d) incidental memory.

5. Hubbard and Seng (1954) said that baseball batters stopped trying to track the ball onto the bat because:

    (a) they relied on the feel of the movement rather than sight,

    (b) it is better to focus on where the ball is going to be hit,

    (c) after a certain time it is too late to alter the shot,

    (d) foveal vision cannot keep track of the ball at high speeds.

6. According to Lee and Young (1985), tau (τ) is:

    (a) the speed at which an object approaches the person,

    (b) the rate at which the retinal image of the object changes size,

    (c) the person's judgement of the rate at which the size of the retinal image is changing,

    (d) the trajectory at which an object approaches the person.

7. The theory of τ was criticized for not taking into account:

(a) changes in the acceleration of the object,

(b) the distance the object has to travel,

(c) the height at which the object is travelling,

(d) individual differences in eyesight.

8. When τ is perceived:

(a) the person then decides what is the best way to intercept the object,

(b) the person automatically responds,

(c) the person will respond if they have past experience of similar situations,

(d) the CNS organizes the response.

Part two

Fill in the blank spaces using words taken from the list below (NB there are more words in the list than there are spaces).

While coincidence anticipation is vital in sports like tennis, _____ and _____, perceptual anticipation is very important in team games. Perceptual anticipation refers to the ability of a performer to predict upcoming events based on _____ _____. There are three main types of perceptual anticipation. _____ is the prediction of where a person thinks an event will occur. _____ anticipation is the timing of an event or when it will happen, while _____ anticipation refers to anticipating what will happen. To the Information Processing theorists, perceptual anticipation is a product of _____ _____. Without past _____ of similar events, we are not able to anticipate. However, they believe that anticipation can be either _____ or _____. Ecological psychologists believe that experience is not essential because all the necessary information is present in the _____. For example in tennis, information from your opponent's _____ and _____ are all you need to anticipate what shot he/she is going to play. Anticipation, however, will be aided by the person becoming _____ ___ _____.

Research into perceptual anticipation originally used a temporal _____ paradigm. Jones and Miles (1978) showed film clips of a tennis player serving to experienced coaches and _____ tennis players. The film was stopped two frames before _____ _____, at contact and two frames after. Experienced players were able to anticipate where the ball would land better than the inexperienced players. Jones and Miles measured the difference between where the ball actually landed and where the participant _____. The amount of error was measured. This is called _____ _____. Jones and Miles' experiment lacked realism because the participants had to mark down on a _____ of the _____ where they thought the ball had landed. Clatworthy, Holder and Graydon (1991) overcame this in a hockey goalkeeping test by having the goalkeepers _____ making a save.

Abernethy and Russell (1987) wanted to know which parts of the display provided the most information. Therefore, they _____ _____ parts of the player's body. Research, using eye-mark recorders, has also tried to determine which areas of the display provide the most information. Eye-mark recorders allow the researcher to see what the participant is _____ _____. Results of this research show that, in ball games, good players can use _____ that are present before the ball has been released, in order to decide where it will land. Most research has measured _____ differences. As expected, experts have been shown to be superior. Little research has examined _____ differences. Learning studies have shown that _____ can be acquired.

time	body	occlusion	event
conscious	working memory	racket	sub-conscious
expert–novice	blocked out	display	map
Spatial	cues	Temporal	lateral error
cricket	experience	constraints	focusing on
inexperienced	explicit	action	anticipation
anticipated	baseball	radial error	simulate
perception	task constraints	racket–ball contact	
expert–intermediate	attuned to affordances	partial information	
court			

Additional reading

Abernethy B (1991) Visual search strategies and decision-making in sport. *Int J Sport Psych* **22**: 189–210

Latham A-M (1997) The use and development of anticipatory skills in netball. *Brit J Phys Educ* **28**: 26–29

6 Memory

Learning Objectives

By the end of this chapter, you should be able to

♦ define memory

♦ understand the nature of the sensory information store, short-term memory and long-term memory

♦ understand the limitations of the sensory information store

♦ understand the limitations of short-term memory and short-term motor memory

♦ understand the factors that affect retention in short-term memory and short-term motor memory

♦ understand the factors that affect retention in long-term memory and long-term motor memory

♦ understand the factors that lead to forgetting in short-term memory and short-term motor memory

♦ understand the factors that lead to forgetting in long-term memory and long-term motor memory

Acquisition and Performance of Sports Skills   T. McMorris
© 2004 John Wiley & Sons, Ltd   ISBNs: 0-470-84994-0 (HB); 0-470-84995-9 (PB)

Introduction

In this chapter we examine what, to the Information Processing theorists, is the basis of their theory, namely *memory*. Tulving (1985) described memory as being the '*capacity that permits organisms to benefit from their past experiences*'. This definition covers all types of memory, e.g., verbal, visual, emotional and motor. In this text, we are interested in verbal and visual memory, especially where they aid decision making and learning. We are, of course also, interested in *motor memory*. Motor memory could be described as *the ability to consistently reproduce a skill over a period of time*. Even ecological psychologists accept that this happens.

Information Processing Theory and memory

As can be seen from Figure 1.4, memory plays a part in the decision-making process and in learning. We have discussed the role of memory in decision making in Chapter 3, so we will not spend time on it here. The main part of this chapter will examine memory with regard to the way in which we learn and is, therefore, linked to Chapter 8. We will look at the sub-divisions of memory, the sensory information store, STM, LTM and motor memory.

Before beginning this, we should point out that the CNS *does not have a specific area which can be described as 'the' memory*. Rather memory is a complicated inter-relationship between different areas in the brain. Memory is developed by links being made between neurons in the CNS. These may be within one part of the brain, e.g., the sensory cortex, or may be between different parts of the brain, e.g., the sensory and motor cortices. It *takes time* for these inter-connections to be made. *Not just time while we are actively learning but also when we have finished overtly learning*, e.g., when resting or even sleeping. The formation of inter-connections or inter-wiring within the CNS is sometimes described as the laying down of *engrams*.

Sensory information store

Not all Information Processing theorists subscribe to the existence of a *sensory information store (SIS)*. This is particularly so with regard to motor memory. Those that accept the existence of the SIS argue that all incoming information is held for a brief time in the SIS. Most of the information is lost *within 0.5 s*. It is only retained and processed if it is *attended to*. This you will recall is similar to what we covered with regard to selective attention in Chapter 2. The retained information is the selectively attended to stimuli. If this information is to pass to STM, it must be *rehearsed*. I do not like the use of the word rehearsal, with regard to memory, but we will come across it again. To most people rehearsal includes a physical element. In these terms it does not necessarily, although it could do. Rehearsal really means being attended to, or processed mentally and/ or physically.

Short-term memory

Whether you believe that information from the environment proceeds through the SIS to the STM or whether information has direct access to STM, it is generally agreed that the STM has a *limited capacity*. This limitation is in both *time* and *space*. Ninety per cent of all information entering the STM is lost within 10 s. Retention and passage to the LTM are dependent on rehearsal – mental or physical or both. Rehearsal occurs naturally around the age of 9 years. It can be used prior to that age but only if the child is told to use it. The instinctive use of rehearsal can be seen when we try to remember telephone numbers. We repeat what we are told. As a child, I can vividly remember running to the shops repeating what I had to buy over and over again so that I would not forget. We can also see instances of rehearsal in physical education classes. Watch the children when they are waiting their turn to try out a skill that they have just been shown. You will see many of them physically making the movements.

Perhaps the most important limitation on STM is one of *capacity* or *space*. Miller (1953) carried out an experiment in which he gave people information to remember. He found that individuals could remember 7 ± 2 bits of information. Later research with children showed that it is much lower for them, e.g., 12-year olds have a span of no more than 5 bits and 7-year olds 3 bits. If Miller were literally correct, my errands to the shop, as a child, would have been limited to less than nine items. Similarly, we would not be able to remember telephone numbers of more than nine digits or repeat a sentence with more than nine words. Commonsense tells us that we can. Get someone to show you a list of 15 numbers. Try to learn them. Give yourself about 20 s. Then try to repeat them. I will be very surprised if you only managed nine. So Miller must be wrong – well not necessarily.

What strategy did you use to try to remember the numbers? Did you group them into twos or threes or fours? Using these strategies is called *chunking*. Not a very scientific sounding word but a good description of what we actually do. Instinctive chunking starts at about 7 years of age. Children younger than that can use chunking but only if shown how. When we chunk, we are in essence making *each chunk 1 bit of information*. So if you chunked in threes, you only held 5 bits of information not 15. We can see this when we learn songs or poetry. We learn phrases rather than single words. A method of aiding STM, similar to chunking, is *labelling*. When we label, we give a chunk of information a name or label. Giving a name to a Rugby scrum makes it easier for us to remember the positions of the individual players. So we hold one bit of information in STM but there are 16 players in the scrum.

Using the examples I have given above, it is easy to define a chunk but I have difficulty in deciding what constitutes a chunk when the information is visual. In our example, the numbers you had to remember can easily be broken into chunks of three or four, but when we watch someone perform a motor skill it is not as easy to break the parts down into chunks. If you used chunks of three, when remembering the numbers, you had 5 bits of information. However, if you watch someone performing an Arab spring and flick-flack, how many chunks and bits did you use? Unfortunately, I do not have an answer nor am I aware of any research which has examined this problem.

When I coach, I try to help the person break the information down into chunks. For example, when I introduce kicking a soccer ball to beginners I try to break it down into the approach, position of non-kicking foot, point of foot–ball contact and follow through – 4 bits of information? I am not certain. What I am certain of is that some children cannot handle that amount of information, even when their developmental stage suggests that 4 bits is well within their capacity.

Forgetting in short-term memory

If rehearsal is necessary for retention in STM and passage to LTM then obviously a lack of rehearsal will result in forgetting. The point of interest to us, therefore, is how and why would the person fail to rehearse. A failure to rehearse may be due to the individual paying no attention to the information. This may be because they do not perceive the information as being important.

The main cause of individuals failing to rehearse or process important information is *overloading*. Overloading refers to situations when the amount of information to be rehearsed is greater than the individual's STM capacity. As we saw earlier, the person can overcome this to some extent by using chunking and labelling but the chunks still need to be within the person's capacity.

Moreover, when faced with novel material it can be very difficult for the individual to chunk or label. The example of labelling I gave, above, was a Rugby scrum. It is easy to label this if one knows something about Rugby. To the uninitiated it can look to be, what in fact it is, a mass of intertwined bodies. Similarly, it is easy to chunk when there are easily recognizable sub-groups to what has to be remembered. North American telephone numbers are a good example of this. They are given in three chunks – the state code (three numbers), the area code (three numbers) and the person's individual number (four numbers). However, as I stated earlier, trying to chunk visual information can be far more difficult.

I watched one of my students trying to teach the cricket bowling action to someone who had never played cricket and had only seen it played, briefly, on television. He gave an excellent demonstration of how to bowl and asked her to repeat what he had done. Although she had watched intently, when she tried to copy his action she only managed the run up. She then stopped, totally fazed. There was simply too much information for her. When it was broken down, she learnt quickly and in a very short space of time was bowling legally and fairly accurately. I doubt that the number of chunks that the young lady was expected to remember actually stretched her STM capacity. She simply did not know enough about the game to be able to determine what bits could be divided into chunks.

I stated above that when I was coaching beginners to kick a ball in soccer I tried to help them to chunk by breaking the skill down into four parts – the approach, the position of the non-kicking foot at the time of contact, the point of foot–ball contact and the follow through. Despite this, I often had to break the skill down even further especially with young children whose STM capacity may well have been below four bits. Nevertheless, I have often heard coaches say to youngsters: 'We are going to learn how to kick a ball. First, you run up to the ball, with a curved run. When you reach the ball, place your non-kicking foot alongside the ball. Swing your kicking leg through and make contact with the ball using your instep. In order to keep the ball down, make sure that you kick the ball through its mid-point. Keep your knee and body over the ball. Follow through in the line that you want the ball to go. Maintain your balance by spreading your arms.' Then they wonder why the children cannot do it.

The second major factor stopping the person from rehearsing is when there is *interference between the exposure to the information and the time to repeat it.* This is particularly important in short-term motor memory (STMM) and is dealt with in detail in the next section. However, it does also happen with verbal and visual information.

Try it for yourself. Get someone to write down a series of numbers, as we did earlier. Learn them and repeat them immediately. Then do the same (using different numbers) but this time copy the first three lines of this paragraph onto a piece of paper. Then try to recall the numbers. You can, also, repeat the second part of this little experiment but this time say your eight times table before trying to repeat the numbers. This will probably cause even more disruption because of its similarity to the information you were asked to repeat.

Short-term motor memory

Far less is known about STMM than STM. It is obviously easier to carry out research into visual and verbal STM than it is STMM. The majority of research into STMM has examined time limitations. There is some controversy about the amount of time that can go between performing the movement once and repeating it for a second time, without significant loss of memory. This period of time is known as the *retention interval*. It is unanimously accepted that *the greater the retention interval the greater the amount of forgetting*. It should be stressed, however, that this is not necessarily a linear relationship and can be very individual. For most people, it is thought that *after about 80 s there is almost complete forgetting*.

The source of the contention between researchers is at the other end of the spectrum, namely examining the length of time before significant forgetting is first registered. An estimate, based on the research literature, would suggest that loss of memory begins after 20 to 30 s. Although it may appear strange that psychologists cannot decide more definitively on a time, there is a good reason for this. As you will remember from the beginning of this chapter, rehearsal does not only mean physical rehearsal, it can be mental. Therefore, if the person is using mental rehearsal, forgetting will be less than if they are not. The problem for researchers is how do they know what the individual is thinking about during the retention interval. Many researchers have tried to ensure that the person does not mentally rehearse the movement by giving them something else to do during the retention intervals, just as I did when I asked you to remember numbers. This may appear to be a sound method but it, in itself, causes another problem. What we ask the person to do during the retention period is called *interpolated activity* and we know that it can disrupt memory. Think back to what happened to you when I asked you to copy out some writing or say your eight times table. So the researcher is left not knowing, for sure, whether the problem is simply a time factor or an interference factor.

A simple way of examining how physical interpolated activity can hinder motor memory is to close your eyes and draw a line. Ask someone to place your hand back at the start of the line and try to re-draw it. Measure the amount of error. Then do the same again except this time repeatedly touch the top then the bottom of the page with your pencil, as quickly as you can. Do this for 20 s. Then try to re-draw the line.

Interference in STMM is, however, even more complicated than that stated above. If we are trying to repeat a new skill we can suffer from *proactive interference* or *inhibition*. This is when a previously learned skill disrupts our recall of the new skill. It is a particular problem if the two skills are similar to one another. A good example is a tennis player learning the forehand in squash. There are some similarities between the two shots but there are also differences. Nevertheless, we often see the tennis player become confused or end up playing a tennis shot. I personally had problems with this when learning to play a backhand in tennis. I had played a great deal of table tennis before learning tennis and found myself playing backhand flicks instead of a tennis backhand. This is not to be recommended, as the wrist is not strong enough to play a backhand flick to a tennis ball travelling at speed.

The learning of a new skill may in turn affect the performance of a previously learned skill. This is called *retroactive interference* or *inhibition*. This will only happen if the old skill has not been learnt to any great extent. It can be seen in many physical education classes, however. For example, the teacher has the children practice putting the shot and then teaches them to throw a discus. When they return to putting the shot there is often retroactive inhibition. If the old skill is well learnt, however, retroactive inhibition will not occur. Learning to play tennis had no effect on my playing of table tennis, as the shots I played in table tennis had become automatic.

As you can see, most of the research into STMM has been concerned with forgetting rather than remembering. What has been examined from a remembering perspective has been whether we retain distances moved better than we do the location to which we have moved. Close your eyes and draw a line. Move your hand to a different location and try to draw the same length of line. Then draw another line and have a friend move your hand back to a point nearer to or further away from the location you ended at, but along the same axis. Try to take your pencil back to where you finished. Do both several times and calculate the mean error. Which was the more accurate, distance or location? Research has almost unequivocally shown location to be remembered better than distance.

It is difficult to know to what extent this type of research has any ecological validity. I suppose it is not too dissimilar to learning to play a drive in golf. If the person can remember the location at the top of the backswing, at the point of contact and at the end of the swing, this must help him/her play the shot. In more open skills, where one cannot dictate the start and contact points, it may have less relevance.

Long-term memory

We have previously discussed the role of LTM in making decisions, therefore in this chapter, we will concentrate on its role in learning. According to the Information Processing theorists, something is learned when it is permanently stored in LTM. The development of a LTM store is the aim of learning. Unlike STM, LTM has *no capacity limitations*. When we think of the vast amount of information we hold this becomes obvious. Just think of how many people's names and faces you can remember. How many songs you know or how many sports performers you can name. In terms of long-term motor memory (LTMM) look at the number of skills you can perform. According to Information Processing Theory these are all held in your LTM or LTMM.

While Information Processing theorists are unanimous in their beliefs concerning the capacity limitations of LTM and LTMM, there is some disagreement about the nature of forgetting. To many there is no such thing as forgetting in LTM or LTMM, *once an engram has been formed*. The inability to recall something is looked upon as being temporary and given time the person will remember. Freud claimed that sometimes we cannot remember because subconsciously we do not wish to. This is not a matter of concern for this book but is a factor worth examining in a sports psychology text. Other Information Processing theorists claim that we do, in fact, forget. They follow the *'use it or lose it'* school of thought. If a skill is not used or a piece of visual or verbal information not recalled regularly, the engram will *decay*. The speed and amount of decay will depend on the *degree of original learning*. The more and better something has been learned, the better and longer it will be remembered. Skills such as riding a bicycle and swimming are often pointed to as examples of activities that we do not forget. We get a good example of remembering visual information when we look at old photographs. We remember the faces of the people we knew well, often remember the faces of others but cannot put names to the faces, but sometimes we do not recognize someone. These latter individuals are normally people we did not know very well.

Another area of disagreement among Information Processing theorists is the way in which information is stored. As we have seen, it is generally accepted that engrams are formed by inter-connections between CNS neurons. This is not in dispute, but the form of storage within the engram is. To some, storage is totally *abstract*. When we recall it, working memory transforms it into visual and/or verbal representations. To others we store visual and motor information visually. We 'see' ourselves or others performing an act. We may not be able to articulate this information. Others think that the CNS stores motor skills in the form of proprioceptive information, allowing us to 'feel' the movement. Many believe that we use a combination of visual, verbal and proprioceptive (feel).

Our desire to visualize motor skills, when they are presented to us verbally, is used to support the notion of motor and visual information being held visually. It has been claimed that we also verbalize information that is presented to us visually. So that we, in fact, have the 'best of both worlds', i.e., we store information verbally and visually. The roles of the different hemispheres of the brain are often pointed at to support this argument. We store visual representations in the right hemisphere and verbal in the left. In remembering, the CNS integrates the visual and the verbal. If perception requires integration of sensory information then it could be argued that memory does the same. Although, at this time, this may appear to be a purely academic argument, in Chapter 8 we will see how it may affect the nature of the type of instruction used when teaching skills

Recall in long-term motor memory

When we examined recall from STM and STMM, we looked at how well the person could *retain* information over a short period of time. The efficiency of this is measured by the amount of discrepancy between the original information and that recalled. Recall from LTM is measured in the same way except that the period of time is greater. Those of you who are studying for examinations will have your ability to recall from LTM tested, when you sit the examinations. Recall in LTMM, however, has some characteristics which are unique. The way in which we measure recall from LTMM is by the amount of the skill which can be repeated following a comparatively long gap between attempts to perform the skill. This is called *retention*. Retention has been described as the *'persistence of a skill over a period of no practice'* (Kerr, 1982).

However, no matter how well we have learned a motor skill *we cannot repeat it totally accurately every time*. This is in contrast to verbal skills or visual information. Once I had learned to recognize someone doing an Arab spring I never made the mistake of saying that it was something else. Similarly, once I had learned that $6 \times 6 = 36$, I never said it was equal to 35 or 37. Yet even when we are expert at performing a motor skill, we do not repeat it perfectly every time. Tiger Woods does not *always* sink 2 m putts. Venus Williams does not always hit her forehand drive within the court and so on. We should be aware that *retention of motor skills is subject to fluctuations in performance.* More surprising than this though is the phenomenon of *reminiscence.* Reminiscence refers to an *improvement in performance over a period of no practice.* You may recall that, in the first paragraph of this chapter, we looked at the fact that the laying down of engrams often took time and so we appear to be learning even when resting after practice. This may be one of the causes of the phenomenon of reminiscence. Another may be that during practice the learner becomes bored or, to put it more scientifically, is affected by *reactive inhibition.* Thus, although they are learning, it is not shown in their performance. Having a break allows the reactive inhibition to dissipate and learning is demonstrated by an improvement in performance.

Another strange factor with regard to LTMM is *overlearning.* As we stated earlier, retention in LTMM does not behave in the same way as retention in LTM. It appears that, even when we have learned a skill, we need to go on practising it. This is called overlearning. It seems that, with motor memory, it is easier to forget than with verbal or visual memory. This may be because, with motor memory, the PNS and CNS are involved, unlike visual and verbal memory where the CNS is solely responsible.

The final unique factor in LTMM to be considered is what is known as the *patterning phenomenon.* Research has consistently shown that *what we forget first is the timing* of a movement rather than the sequencing and spatial organization. However, it is very quickly restored. I had a break of 10 years from playing competitive table tennis. On returning to the game, there was no problem with the organization of the movement patterns except for the timing. I was either too early or too late. Some of my topspin drives did not only miss the table but went over my opponents' heads. Those of you who play seasonal games like tennis or cricket or baseball may well have experienced timing problems at the beginning of a season.

Ecological psychology and attunement to affordances

Initially ecological psychologists did not accept that past experiences, other than developmental changes, affected performance at all. The evidence for experience changing performance, however, forced a rethink. As a result, the notion of attunement to affordances came about. They argued that repeated exposure to an environment increases the individual's ability to recognize affordances. However, they claimed that this is not a form of memory.

Dynamical Systems theorists believe that memory plays a part in the choosing of goals, which determine the affordances. It plays no other part.

Many Information Processing theorists find the claim that 'attunement to affordances is not a form of memory' unacceptable. To the ecological psychologists, however, it is not a form of memory because it does not require the recall of past performance in order to achieve the desired goal. To the ecological psychologists, attunement to affordances is not due to the formation of engrams within the CNS. It is simply the triggering off of possible perception–action couplings. These are not inter-connected physically, in the CNS or PNS, but simply facilitate the recognition of the affordance. The relationship is similar to the Information Processing theorists' claim that familiar stimuli can be processed more quickly than unfamiliar stimuli. This aspect of ecological psychology theory is, for most people, the most difficult to understand or accept. There is undoubtedly a lack of clarity about what is meant by attunement to affordances.

Key points

- Memory is the capacity that permits us to benefit from past experiences (Tulving, 1985).

- Motor memory is the persistence of a skill over a period of time.

Sensory information store

- All incoming information is held for a very brief period:
  - information is lost within 0.5 s, unless it is rehearsed,
  - rehearsed information is passed to the short-term memory,
  - SIS may not exist for motor memory.

Short-term memory

- STM has a limited capacity in terms of time and space:
  - all information is lost within 10 s, unless it is rehearsed,

- o   it can only deal with 7 ± 2 bits of information.

- Capacity problems can be overcome, to some extent, by the use of:

  - o   chunking (grouping together information to form chunks – each chunk becomes one bit of information),

  - o   labelling (giving information or chunks names).

- Retention is dependent upon:

  - o   rehearsal (rehearsed information is retained and passed to long-term memory),

  - o   rehearsal can be physical and/or mental.

- Forgetting occurs through:

  - o   failing to rehearse,

  - o   overloading (having to remember more than 7 ± 2 bits),

  - o   interference between exposure to the information and the need to repeat it.

Short-term motor memory

- Rehearsal:

  - o   information that is not rehearsed is lost within 80 s,

  - o   rehearsal can be physical and/or mental,

  - o   the greater the length of the retention interval, the greater the amount of forgetting.

- Forgetting is due to:

  - o   interpolated activity (activity between exposure and recall),

  - o   proactive inhibition (a previously-learned skill affects the performance of a new skill),

  - o   retroactive inhibition (the learning of a new skill affects the performance of an old-learned skill; this will only occur if the old skill is not well learned).

Long-term memory

- LTM has no capacity limitations.
- Forgetting:
  - some argue that there is no forgetting in long-term memory,
  - some follow the argument that information will be lost unless we use it (decay theory),
  - the degree of original learning will affect whether we forget or not.

Long-term motor memory

- Retention is the persistence of a skill over a period of no practice.

- Reminiscence is an improvement in performance following a period of no practice.

- Retention is aided by overlearning (continuing to practise even after the skill has been learnt).

- Forgetting is affected by the patterning phenomenon:
  - sequencing and spatial organization are retained better than timing.

Ecological psychology and attunement to affordances

- Experience and practice aid performance:
  - we become attuned to affordances.

Test your knowledge

(Answers in Appendix 3.)

Part one

Choose which of the phrases, (a), (b), (c) or (d), best completes the statement or answers the question. There is only *one* correct answer for each problem.

1. Most information will be lost from the sensory information store within:

    (a) 0.5 s,

    (b) 1.0 s,

    (c) 1.5 s,

    (d) 2.0 s.

2. Some Information Processing theorists believe that the sensory information store does not exist for:

    (a) complex skills,

    (b) continuous skills,

    (c) fine motor skills,

    (d) all motor skills.

3. For adults, short-term memory has a capacity limitation of:

    (a) 4 ± 2 bits of information,

    (b) 5 ± 2 bits of information,

    (c) 6 ± 2 bits of information,

    (d) 7 ± 2 bits of information.

4. For a 13-year old, short-term memory has a capacity limitation of:

    (a) 4 ± 2 bits of information,

    (b) 5 ± 2 bits of information,

(c) 6 ± 2 bits of information,

(d) 7 ± 2 bits of information.

5. Ninety per cent of information entering short-term memory is lost within:

(a) 5 s,

(b) 10 s,

(c) 15 s,

(d) 20 s.

6. Spontaneous rehearsal occurs at about:

(a) 7 years old,

(b) 8 years old,

(c) 9 years old,

(d) 10 years old.

7. In short-term motor memory, if the skill is not repeated there will be complete forgetting within:

(a) 50 s,

(b) 60 s,

(c) 70 s,

(d) 80 s.

8. When the performance of an old skill is disrupted by a new skill, we are said to be exhibiting:

(a) proactive facilitation,

(b) retroactive facilitation,

(c) proactive inhibition,

(d) retroactive inhibition,

9. Storage in long-term memory has:

(a) a capacity limitation of 7 ± 2 bits of information,

(b) a capacity limitation of 5 bits of information,

(c) a capacity limitation of 8 ± 2 bits of information,

(d) no capacity limitation.

10. When a performer maintains his/her level of performance over a period of no practice, it is called:

(a) retention,

(b) reminiscence,

(c) patterning phenomenon,

(d) overlearning.

11. When a performer shows an improvement in performance over a period of no practice, this is called:

(a) retention,

(b) reminiscence,

(c) patterning phenomenon,

(d) overlearning.

12. The first part of a skill to be forgotten is:

(a) timing,

(b) spatial organization,

(c) sequencing,

(d) patterning.

Part two

Which of the following statements are true (T) and which are false (F)?

1.   There is no such thing as a part of the brain called memory.   T   F

2.	Motor memory is the persistence of a skill over a period of time.	T	F
3.	Information held in the sensory information store can enter short-term memory even if it is not attended to.	T	F
4.	Children aged 5 years old automatically use chunking.	T	F
5.	Children aged 5 years old automatically use labelling.	T	F
6.	Overloading causes forgetting in short-term memory.	T	F
7.	Interpolated activity is activity between exposure to information and having to repeat the information.	T	F
8.	Retroactive inhibition is unlikely to occur if the old skill has been well learned.	T	F
9.	With motor skills, we remember distance moved better than the location moved to.	T	F
10.	The degree of original learning has no effect on retention in long-term memory.	T	F
11.	Proprioceptive retention of information means we 'see' ourselves doing the skill.	T	F
12.	Engrams are inter-connections between neurons in the CNS.	T	F
13.	Continuing to practise a skill once it has been learned aids long-term motor memory.	T	F
14.	According to Dynamical Systems theorists, we do not hold information in memory but simply become attuned to affordances.	T	F

Additional reading

Allard F and Burnett N (1985) Skill in sport. *Can J Psych* **39**: 294–312

Fischman MG, Christina RW and Vercuyssen MJ (1981) Retention and transfer of motor skills: A review for the practitioner. *Quest* **33**: 181–194

7 Motor Control

Learning Objectives

By the end of this chapter, you should be able to

♦ understand the nature and role of proprioception

♦ understand how Information Processing Theory explains how we move, with reference to

◊ efferent organization

◊ motor programs

◊ role of the PNS

◊ role of feedforward

◊ role of feedback

♦ understand how Dynamical Systems Theory explains how we move, with reference to

◊ self-organization

◊ role of the CNS

◊ role of the PNS

◊ effect of constraints on movement

◊ visual guidance of movement

♦ understand some of the basic strengths and weaknesses of each of the theories

Acquisition and Performance of Sports Skills   T. McMorris
© 2004 John Wiley & Sons, Ltd   ISBNs: 0-470-84994-0 (HB); 0-470-84995-9 (PB)

Introduction

While ecological psychologists have received a great deal of criticism for their claims about the role of memory in performance, in this chapter we examine the subject which has led to the most criticism for Information Processing theorists, namely motor control. Moreover, just as ecological psychologists have reorganized their thinking about memory, by accepting that the individual can become attuned to affordances, the Information Processing theorists have been forced to rethink their explanations of motor control. Both schools accept that there are roles in motor control for both the CNS and PNS; however, their relative importance and what they actually do are sources of great debate.

Before examining the theory of motor control, I think we should pause for a moment to ponder what it is we are talking about when we talk of motor control. Motor control refers to the way in which we are able, repeatedly, to perform motor skills, both simple (if there is such a thing) and complex. The range and difficulty of skills performed by human beings never fails to amaze me. We have become blasé about what humans can do. Watching ice skating on television, I heard the commentator say, 'oh dear, she could only manage a double Salchow' – only! I know what he meant. If you are to get to the top in ice skating you will need to do a triple Salchow, but if we think about what is necessary to do 'just' a single Salchow we realize how skilled people are. Personally, I would love to be able to skate without feeling the need to be near the sides of the rink.

Double and triple Salchows are, of course, complex skills and only the elite can perform them. However, there are many skills which we consider simple which in fact, require a great deal of co-ordination. As I am typing this – a skill in itself (thank goodness for spell checks) – if I look out of my window I can see a workman balancing on a ladder while cutting a branch off a tree. I am sure that the workman does not see himself as being very skilful, but in fact what he is doing requires balance, whole body co-ordination, visual perception, co-ordination of his arm movements and power in his arm. Just think of how many groups of muscles are involved. A good example from sport would be swimming the breaststroke. The co-ordination of movement and the timing of that co-ordination require a lot of control. Even walking is a none too easy skill. Watch a baby learning to walk and you get some idea of the problems. We take walking for granted because we do not remember learning to do it. Moreover, it is now automatic to us, therefore we do not see it as being difficult. That does not mean that it is not difficult. To the expert ice skater a triple Salchow is not too difficult but we, mere mortals, know that it is.

Information Processing Theory and motor control

CNS–PNS interaction

There is great controversy about the interaction between the CNS and PNS in the control of movement. In this section, we will examine neuropsychological evidence. In the following sections, emphasis will change to theoretical explanations. As you will see, however, even the neuropsychological 'evidence' is incomplete and affected by interpretation.

Technological advances in electromyographs (EMG), electroencephalographs (EEG) and magnetic resonance imaging (MRI) have allowed us to know more about what happens in the CNS and PNS during physical activity. Although, this information is far from complete, it is generally accepted that voluntary movements are initiated by the *premotor cortex*. The information is passed to the primary motor cortex, the basal ganglia and the cerebellum. What exactly the *primary motor cortex* does is one of the main areas of debate and has been since the early work of Sherrington, almost 100 years ago.

The premotor cortex sends information to the basal ganglia and cerebellum as well as the primary motor cortex. These in turn pass the information to the brain stem and hence to the spinal cord. The *basal ganglia* are thought to be responsible for the regulation of movements of shorter than one reaction time but not longer movements. They receive no feedback from the PNS amd therefore are not capable of amending ongoing movements. The *cerebellum*, on the other hand, is thought to be mainly responsible for the control of movements of greater than one reaction time, as it receives information directly from the PNS. It probably also plays a part in the regulation of shorter movements, as it receives the same information from the CNS as do the basal ganglia.

The information received by the basal ganglia and the cerebellum, from the premotor cortex, is thought to be about the intended movement. The interaction between the motor cortex and these areas of the brain are believed to refine the CNS instructions to make sure that the neural messages to the brain stem are those that were intended. This is known as *feedforward*. The cerebellum also monitors feedback from the PNS to regulate ongoing movements and to make alterations where necessary, so that the intended action takes place. Figure 7.1 provides an outline of this process in diagrammatic form.

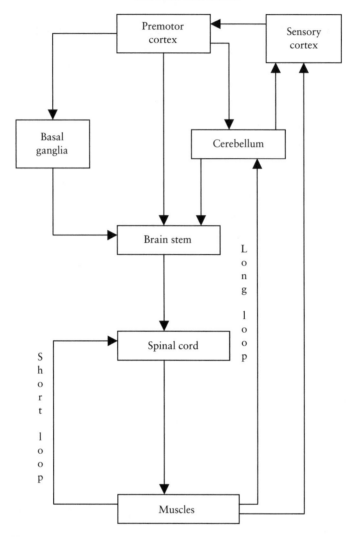

Figure 7.1 Interaction between the CNS and PNS when controlling movement

Proprioception

The information coming from the higher centres of the brain is passed down to
the muscles by *efferent nerves* or *motoneurons* in the spinal cord and information from the muscles is returned to the CNS by *afferent* or *sensory neurons*,
also situated in the spinal cord. This sensory information has been given the
name *proprioception*. Proprioception is a form of perception, but it is more
than that. Both ecological psychologists and Information Processing theorists
agree that it not only detects movement but also helps control it. Strictly
speaking proprioception is the *perception of the body and its position in space*

(Sherrington, 1906). The term *kinaesthesis* (or kinesthesis) was used to describe the person's perception of the movements of his/her whole body and separate body parts. As you can see the definitions of proprioception and kinaesthesis are very similar and have become so intertwined that today they are used to describe the same phenomenon – *the individual's ability to know where his/her body is in space and to be aware of the positions of the different limbs.*

Visual proprioception

The phrase *visual proprioception* was coined by the ecological psychologists. To the linguists among you it will appear to be a contradiction of terms. The Latin root of proprioception, *'proprio'*, means inside one's body, while vision, of course, is concerned with factors outside of the body. However, if we look at our definition of proprioception, the person is concerned with knowledge coming from within their body (i.e., awareness of the position of limbs) and from outside of the body (i.e., where the body is in space). Vision will, of course, provide much information about the latter but it also provides invaluable information about the former. The ability to see where your limbs are aids perception of their position and movement. The real importance of vision to aid proprioception, however, is only just being discovered.

As we saw in Chapter 2, there are two types of vision, foveal and ambient. Both play important roles in visual proprioception but the latter is probably the more important. The role of horizontal peripheral vision to aid balance has been recognized for some time. While balancing, horizontal *and* vertical peripheral vision provide us with information about our position with reference to the floor, the roof or sky, walls or trees and buildings. All of this information is valuable in helping us discern whether or not we are upright. A simple test of the use of vision while balancing is to stand on one foot with your eyes open. Focus attention on your ankles. How much work do they have to do to maintain balance? Then repeat the task with your eyes closed. You will undoubtedly feel a dramatic difference. Even blind people sway more than sighted individuals. This may be surprising, as you would think that they would be able to compensate for the loss of sight with better use of their vestibular apparatus compared with sighted people. In fact, they probably can and do use their vestibular apparatus better than sighted people but not sufficiently to make up totally for the lack of vision.

Vision plays roles in far more than balance. It aids our awareness of where our limbs are positioned. Coaches in some sports get their performers to practice blindfolded. The aim is to increase non-visual proprioception. The amount of disruption caused is considerable. Try this simple test. Place three 15 cm squares on the ground in a triangle, about 15 cm apart. In 30 s tap your foot in a triangular pattern and touch each square as many times as possible. Get someone to count how many you touch. Then repeat blindfold. It sounds easy but it is not.

There is no doubt that vision provides a great deal of information concerning awareness of the position of our bodies, body parts and our orientation in space. One of the most graphic examples of how vision affects awareness of the position of our bodies in space comes from aircraft crashes. Pilots in small aircraft, without the navigation aids of commercial aircraft, can become totally disoriented when visibility is reduced. Pilots report that they were unable to tell which way was up and which down. These pilots were the lucky ones who guessed correctly. Deep-sea divers have also described experiencing this kind of disorientation.

The eyes do not only provide exteroceptive information, they can tell us a great deal about head position. This occurs in the *oculomotor system* and in particular its interaction with the vestibular apparatus, this is known as the *vestibulo–oculomotor reflex*. The main purpose of this reflex is to stabilize the image on the retina during active movement. When moving we try to keep the image on the fovea. This is done by *smooth pursuit* in slow movements and by *saccades* in fast movement. In order to do this we must be aware, not only of the visual information but also the vestibular. Thus, we are aware of the position of our body with regard to space. The control of saccades is undertaken by the *prefrontal eye field*, which is not part of the CNS but is adjacent to the *optic nerve*. As a result, some authors have described the optic nerve as being more CNS than PNS. This is not strictly correct but does account to some extent for the speed at which we can respond to visual changes. The efferent or motoneurons in the eye can respond at velocities over two and a half times faster than the motoneurons in the spinal cord. This, in itself, shows the importance of visual proprioception.

Vestibular apparatus

In the last section, we alluded to the vestibular apparatus when talking about the oculomotor–vestibular reflex. The *vestibular apparatus* is located in the inner ear. It is generally spoken about as being responsible for balance, but it has more roles than that. As we have already seen, it provides valuable information about head position, particularly when the information is integrated with visual information. It also tells us much about the speed and direction in which we are moving.

The main structures of the vestibular apparatus are the saccules, utricles and semi-circular canals. The *saccules* and *utricles* provide information concerning the position of the head, with reference to the line of gravity – particularly important to divers and gymnasts. The *semi-circular canals* provide information concerning the direction of movement and changes in acceleration. Very important for dynamic balance as found in many sports, e.g., ice-skating.

Spinal cord and motor control

Until recently it was thought that, in order to regulate ongoing movements, information from the PNS went first to the *sensory cortex* in the CNS. The sensory cortex and the premotor cortex then interacted to alter the commands, so that changes in the movement could be made. Many believed that for simple movements this could be done (but to a limited extent) by the cerebellum. Recent research has supported the assumption that the cerebellum plays a role, possibly a large role, in the regulation of ongoing movements.

Research by Dewhurst (1967) supported this claim. Dewhurst had his participants push a lever against a resistance. At a time unknown to the participant the resistance was increased. EMGs were used to measure the activity of the muscles in the forearm. Between 50 and 80 ms after the resistance was increased there was a burst of activity. This is too short for the information to have been dealt with by the higher centres of the CNS, the sensory and motor cortices, so could only have been controlled by the cerebellum. This is called *long-loop* feedback. There was a later burst of activity some 120–180 ms from increasing the resistance. This would fall inline with a normal reaction time and was almost certainly dealt with by the higher centres of the CNS. It was not *until this time that the participants were aware of having increased the power of their movement.*

This research also demonstrated an even earlier burst of EMG activity, coming only 30 ms after the resistance was increased. This activity can only be explained by a phenomenon called *alpha–gamma* $(\alpha-\gamma)$ *co-activation*. This is sometimes called *short-loop* feedback. This interaction has been known about for a great deal of time but was originally thought of as only being used when there was risk of injury or other physical danger. In school textbooks of the 1950s and 1960s it was referred to as a reflex arc and was normally accompanied by a picture of someone putting their hand into a Bunsen burner flame then withdrawing it quickly. More recently, it has become accepted that the spinal cord is able to respond to a variety of neural inputs and through afferent–efferent interactions regulate more than just movements to avoid danger. This ability of the spinal cord to regulate movement has led to it being dubbed the *smart* spinal cord.

The *spinal cord* is located in the spinal column and is the main route for transmitting nerve impulses to and from the brain. It not only contains motoneurons and afferent neurons but also interneurons, which connect the motoneurons and afferent neurons. The motoneurons responsible for directly exciting muscle are the α motoneurons. The CNS passes information to the muscles, via the α motoneurons, to 'tell' them what to do. It also informs the muscle spindles, sensory nerves within the muscles, what tension they should 'feel' while the muscles are activated. This information is carried by the γ motoneurons. If the muscle spindles perceive the tension to be incorrect, they report this to the spinal cord. The information is evaluated and the α motoneurons issue new commands, so that the correct movement is carried out. This is the $\alpha–\gamma$ co-activation process.

That $\alpha–\gamma$ co-activation exists is just as well. Think about what happens when you 'go over' on your ankle. The information transmitted to the muscles by the α motoneurons has activated a movement. For some reason, possibly uneven terrain, the movement is inappropriate and your ankle begins to buckle. If this information had to be transmitted all the way back to the CNS, you would almost certainly break your ankle. However, because of $\alpha–\gamma$ co-activation, the problem can be dealt with at spinal-cord level thus allowing a re-adjustment in a much shorter period of time.

Muscle spindles are not the only nerve fibres to provide impulses to afferent neurons so that movement can be altered. Here we will only cover the main nerves and very briefly. Those wishing to know more can consult any basic neuro-anatomy text. *Golgi tendon organs* are found between muscles and tendons. They provide information about the amount of stretch in a muscle. They also have a protective function in ensuring that the force of the stretch is not so great that the tendon becomes ruptured. Another group of sensory nerves that provides valuable information is the *joint receptors*. They are found in the joint capsules of various limbs. There are two main joint receptors, the *Ruffini end organs* and the *Pacinian corpuscles*. There is some controversy about what information they actually detect but most authors believe that they provide useful information concerning joint position and movement.

Summary

From what we have covered above, we can see that Information Processing theorists perceive movement as being controlled by an interaction between the

CNS and the PNS. The spinal cord is not only a relay station for efferent or motor nerves to pass information to the muscles and for afferent nerves to provide proprioceptive information to the CNS, it also plays a role in regulating movement. To the cognitivists, however, this role is a fairly minor one. The PNS can only ensure that central commands are carried out efficiently. Any alterations are simply to ensure that the muscles are 'obeying' the instructions sent by the CNS. It is the latter which is responsible for organizing the movement. In the next section we examine how this is done.

Efferent organization

The neuropsychological evidence, examined above, has led to the Information Processing theorists developing theories concerning efferent organization or the way in which the CNS controls movement. The explanation of the early Information Processing theorists concerning movement control has become known as *open-loop control*. They believed that the CNS controls all movement. The action to be taken is determined by the decision process and efferent organization is responsible for controlling the muscles and joints. If you look at Figure 1.4, open-loop control would be depicted by the Information Processing model minus the lower feedback loop, i.e., feedback to the perceptual process. The feedback loop to LTM, the upper loop in the model, was considered to be important. The outcome of the action was stored in LTM. If the movement were successful, it would be repeated. If it were unsuccessful, something different would be tried next time. This is still considered to be the way in which movements of less than one reaction time are controlled.

From observation of people performing skills it soon became obvious that movements of greater than one reaction time could be continually altered during the action. In these cases, it was thought that movement was organized by the CNS, the instructions passed to the limbs via the motoneurons in the spinal cord, sensory information fedback to the CNS by the afferent neurons and then alterations could be made. This, of course, is what we covered in the first part of this chapter (see Figure 7.1). This process is called *closed-loop* control. Note that originally it did not include short- and long-loop control, although these are now generally accepted as having important roles to play in controlling movement. Moreover, it was argued that even movements of greater than one reaction time could be performed under open-loop control if they were well learned and had become automatic. When actions are performed in this manner they are said to be controlled by *motor programs*.

Before moving on to consider the nature of motor programs, we should note that some movements are under *joint open- and closed-loop control*. You can experience this for yourself. Take two pieces of paper and place them about 60 cm apart. Place your pen in the centre of one piece of paper. Move your pen, as quickly as you can, to make a mark on the other piece of paper. Now draw a 3 cm square in the centre of the paper you are using as a target. Repeat the movement but this time make a mark within the 3 cm square. If possible, get someone to time each action. When moving to touch the larger target paper, you probably did so in one movement and used open-loop control, no alterations in the chosen movement pattern. When aiming at the 3 cm square, the initial movement was probably fast, open loop, but as you came near to the target you will have slowed and made any alterations necessary to make sure you got your pen inside the square, closed-loop control.

Motor programs

Keele (1968) defined a motor program as being *a set of muscle commands that allow movements to be performed without any peripheral feedback*. (The American spelling of 'programs' is normally used rather than the UK 'programmes', due to the origins of the theory being in the US. You will, however, sometimes see 'programme' being used.). According to Keele, the person sees a movement and stores a *template* or *model of the task* in their LTM. When they practice the skill, they constantly compare the outcome and the nature of the movement with the template. Thus, this stage can be open or closed loop. During practice, *corrections are made until the action matches the template*, then the motor program is established. Keele believes that this process takes place solely in the motor cortex, basal ganglia and cerebellum. It was further thought that several motor programs could be combined to form an *executive motor program*.

Examples of motor programs are basically any skill that you can think of. Hitting a baseball, catching a netball, doing a cartwheel or a somersault are all examples of motor programs. So, too, are more simple tasks like walking or running. Executive motor programs are normally more complex such as doing a triple jump, where we join together a run, a hop, a step and a jump. Or doing a gymnastics sequence where we join together several smaller motor programs, e.g., Arab spring, flick-flak and back somersault.

The evidence that the Information Processing theorists point to for support for the existence of motor programs is that we are able to carry out many acts without thinking about what we are doing. Moreover, these skills are performed smoothly and consistently and they also appear to take up little CNS channel space. There is also a marked difference between our efforts to perform the skill before and after a motor program has been developed.

Although motor program theory has intuitive appeal, even the early Information Processing theorists were aware that it was not without its weaknesses. Classical motor program theory stated that when a motor program was being developed the person stored the *sequencing, timing and range of movement*. Observation of people performing skills, however, showed that motor programs were not always repeated at the same speed. A tennis player hitting the ball may do so slowly or quickly or in between. When doing this the movement of their arm will differ. Information Processing theorists overcame this problem by saying that although the *overall* timing was different, the *relative timing of the different segments remained the same*. In other words, the ratios between the time taken to move the racket back to the starting position, swing through to the point of contact and follow through to the end of the stroke remained the same whether the whole action was fast or slow.

Another problem, with regard to motor programs, was identified by MacNeilage as early as 1970. MacNeilage (1970) was concerned that, as we have a vast range of motor programs, storage of these in the CNS was difficult to explain given the size of the human brain. MacNeilage therefore argued that we do not store the whole movement but the location of key points in the movement, what he termed *targets*. So our tennis player would store the starting position, point of racket–ball contact and the finishing point. How to move from one point to the other would be taken care of automatically.

The problem of how we explain the storage of motor programs became a major issue with Information Processing theorists. We should remember that, at this time, the microchip had not been developed and the notion that a vast amount of information could be held in a small container was difficult to come to terms with. Computers were massive things. A very simple, relatively limited, computer filled a large room. The idea of lots of computers being housed in one room seemed ridiculous. There were other problems related to storage, however, that are still problematic today. The most important is *specificity* of the program. It was generally held that motor programs were specific. Observation of how we perform skills, however, led to psychologists questioning this. When we kick a soccer ball, we do not do it in the same way every time. The position of the ball relative to us, the weather conditions, the distance and height we wish to kick it and so on will all change the motor program required. So, do we store different motor programs for each of these situations?

This question concerned Information Processing theorists for some time.

Richard Schmidt (1975) provided what is still considered to be the best answer to this question. Schmidt was primarily interested in explaining how we developed so many motor programs. He decided that what we learnt was not specific motor programs but rather *generalized rules* or *schemas*. Thus Schmidt's *Schema Theory* was developed. This is covered in some detail in Chapter 8, examining learning. Based on Schema Theory, *generalized motor program* theory was developed. According to this theory, we learn and store the programs as schemas or sets of generalized rules. This allows us to perform the same skill in a variety of conditions and situations. Moreover, because the rules are generalized, we can adapt when faced with novel situations. According to classical motor program theory, we would not be able to improvise, we would only be able to repeat learnt skills. Observation of sports performance shows that we can and do improvise. In fact, performers who are good improvisers generally reach the top of their sport.

Look at Figure 7.2. Here we see a table tennis player playing a topspin drive in three different positions. According to classical motor program theory, he would need three separate motor programs. Generalized motor program theory suggests that he is simply adapting the basic program to each specific set of conditions.

Following the development of Schema Theory, there was something of a lull in theoretical activity among Information Processing theorists. However, research using high-speed film raised another issue. As we saw in Chapter 4, Bootsma and Van Wieringen showed that performers were able to alter the timing of motor programs during execution. Not only was this contrary to early theories concerning the consistency of the ratios between the different parts of a skill, it raised the problem of *how alterations to the movement could be made in less than one reaction time*. The Information Processing theorists believe that the information necessary to allow such control is sent from the motor cortex to the cerebellum and spinal cord in the form of *feedforward*. In other words the higher centres of the CNS inform the cerebellum and spinal cord what to expect. If there is a mismatch between what was expected and what is actually happening, then the alterations are made automatically.

The nature of the instructions from the motor cortex to the spinal cord has been a source of dispute for some time. In 1906, Sherrington asked whether the instructions were 'muscle commands', i.e., they controlled the firing of specific muscles, or 'movement commands', i.e., they controlled overall movement of the limbs, with the PNS determining the specific muscles to be used. This remains an issue of some disagreement among Information Processing theorists.

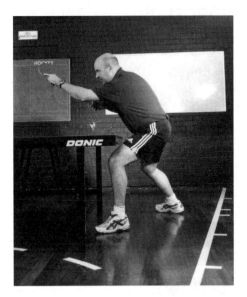
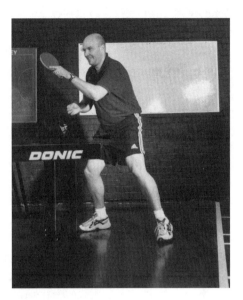
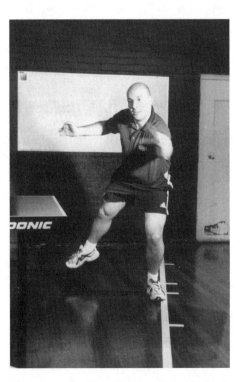

Figure 7.2 Example of a generalized motor program; each shot is a topspin drive but played with different initial conditions and response parameters

Ecological psychology and motor control

While the Information Processing theorists perceive the CNS as being the most important area concerned with motor control, ecological psychologists see it as merely being responsible for *setting the goal* with regard to what the person wishes to do. The CNS decides that we wish to catch a ball or run up a hill or do a cartwheel. The information that the CNS sends to the PNS is not detailed instructions to the muscles, or even instructions concerning the nature of the movement, but rather a *general command*. Such commands are thought to be *functionally specific*. In other words, they are as basic as those I have provided above – 'catch the ball', 'run up the hill', 'do a cartwheel'. Even the instructions concerning the cartwheel would be general rather than specific.

The instructions to 'catch the ball' can be achieved in many different ways depending on the specific situation. The ball may be above our head, down at our feet, or chest high. Each requires different movement patterns in order to catch the ball. That the instruction 'do a cartwheel' is not specific, however, appears to be a contradiction of terms. Surely there is only *one* way to do a cartwheel? This is, in fact, not so. How each person does a cartwheel will be different, depending on their own physical make up and the environment in which they must carry out the task. As you will no doubt remember from Chapter 1, ecological psychologists believe that each skill is affected by constraints. In the case of the cartwheel, the rules concerning the movement are task constraints. There are certain things that must be done for the movement to qualify as a cartwheel. The person's own physical strengths and weaknesses are organismic constraints. Different people will organize their limbs differently, depending on their size, power and flexibility. While the environment will also impose constraints, which are not surprisingly called environmental constraints. For example, doing a cartwheel is different for the gymnast in the gymnasium, in bare feet and on a sprung floor, compared with the professional soccer player doing a cartwheel to celebrate scoring a goal, in soccer boots and on grass.

In Chapter 1, we briefly examined the effect of constraints on motor control. I will elaborate a little on these effects. Task constraints are factors such as rules, e.g., a high jumper takes off from one foot rather than two because the latter is illegal, or a hockey player uses only one side of the stick. A task constraint can also come about because the chosen movement is the most effective for that particular skill, e.g., a golfer, when driving, uses a long swing because the laws of physics have shown that this is the most appropriate method if distance is to be obtained.

As far as environmental constraints are concerned, we know that running on soft sand is very different from running on a tartan running track. Canoeing in calm water requires different movements from canoeing in white water. Some would argue that as far as motor control is concerned, organismic constraints are the most important. Each individual brings their own physical, neuronal and mental conditions to the task. Although the goal may be the same for two people, the way in which they achieve it will be very different. Golfers driving from the tee are a good example. They often have very different movement patterns yet achieve the same result. Bowlers in cricket and pitchers in baseball are also good examples of this. Sometimes different patterns can only be spotted with the use of biomechanical methods of analysis.

That there are differences in the actual movement patterns is brought about because our movement control is *self-organizing*. In describing self-organization, ecological psychologists often explain how different limbs work together. In our example of the cartwheel, the arms and legs work together to produce the movement. The way in which they work together is a result of natural interactions between muscles and joints. When the person alters their centre of gravity, at the beginning of the cartwheel, other limb positions will be automatically controlled due to the laws of mechanics. The muscles and joints will co-ordinate in the way that is the most economic or comfortable for each individual. This is sometimes called the *least-effort principle*.

A good way of seeing how muscles and joints self-organize is to stand on one leg and lean forward. Your other leg automatically moves backwards to stop you falling over. Your arms will normally move outwards to aid your balance. Walk across a gymnastics beam and see how you automatically use your arms to aid balance. Look at out table tennis player in Figure 7.2. Observe the different positions of his right arm and right leg as he stretches to play the topspin drive.

Self-organization at limb level is thought, by ecological psychologists, to answer a question posed by Bernstein. Bernstein was concerned with what he called the degrees of freedom problem. *Degrees of freedom* refer to the number of muscles and joints that need to be co-ordinated when we make a movement. Think of our cartwheel. How many limbs are involved? How many muscles and joints are involved? To the ecological psychologists the development of motor programs, even generalized motor programs, does not explain how we can control so many muscles, joints and nerves. They argue that it is not possible for the CNS to control all these structures. If, however, we look at the body as being made up of many interacting structures, obeying the laws of physics and biology, we can explain the control of so many muscles, joints, afferent and efferent nerves, i.e., degrees of freedom.

The professional dancer and movement expert Len Heppell, who worked with top athletes from many sports in the 1980s, used the basic laws of physics to aid movement. Heppell was consulted by many professional games players to help them improve their ability to turn quickly. Heppell claimed that the key factor in turning was not the legs or lower body but the head! He argued that, as the head is the heaviest single body component, if you begin the turn with your head the rest of the body must follow. The most startling example of this is the gymnastic move called a *'falling leaf'*. Figure 7.3 shows a falling leaf being performed. Once the person throws their head back the rest of their body will naturally follow and swing round to land on the feet. (If you wish to try to perform a falling leaf, only do so with someone who is trained to teach gymnastics. Although the movement is natural, sometimes people try to abort it just after they have begun to fall. This can have dire consequences. Also, if the height of the beam is set incorrectly you can over-rotate, also causing problems. As you can see in Figure 7.3, even our gymnast has used a spotter.)

Although ecological psychologists argue that much of motor control can be explained by the principles of physics and mechanics, they do not rule out short-loop and long-loop control. Ecological psychologists accept that $\alpha-\gamma$ co-activation and control by the cerebellum take place. They even do not rule out control by the motor cortex but believe that motor control is better explained by the self-organization of muscles, joints and nerves.

Visual guidance of movement

Like the Information Processing theorists, the ecological psychologists are adamant that vision is the most important of the senses, even for motor control. As I stated earlier, it was the ecological psychologists who coined the phrase visual proprioception. As well as those areas of visual proprioception covered earlier in this chapter, the ecological psychologists turn to Action Systems Theory to further explain the role of vision in the control of movement. As you will remember from Chapter 1, to the ecological psychologists you can not extract perception from action. The two are intertwined through perception-action coupling. We examined this when, in Chapter 2, we looked at the role of τ in making an interceptive action. In Chapter 2, we concentrated on the perceptual side of the perception–action coupling that τ represents, particularly examining how the movement of the object provides the information necessary to make an interception.

Of particular interest to us in this chapter is the use of τ when we are the moving object and our target is static, as well as when the object is moving. Lee, Lishman and Thomas (1984) examined the former using the long jump as an

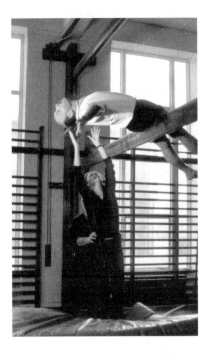
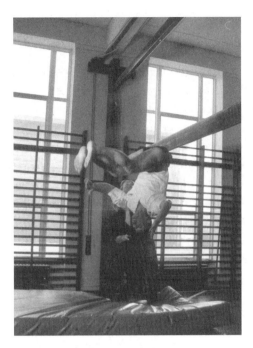
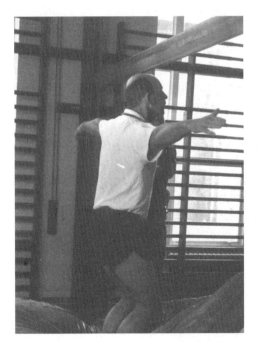

Figure 7.3 The falling leaf, an example of self-organization; once the gymnast has thrown his head backwards, the rest of his body automatically controls his movement

example. Despite the fact that most long jumpers take great care in measuring out their run up, Lee found that the run was uniform until the later stages when the athlete made corrections to try to hit the take-off board. The athletes were not aware of doing this and most certainly did not make a conscious effort to alter their stride pattern. When out jogging, I have noticed myself doing this as I approach kerbs. I automatically alter my stride pattern so that stepping onto the kerb will be as much within my stride as possible (the least-effort principle most definitely applies). Lee pointed out that, even if the athletes measured their run up exactly correctly, once they began running the precision of the measurements would become superfluous because such factors as changes in wind strength and increased effort would mean that the exact stride pattern was lost. Therefore, the athlete will never repeat the same movement, so measuring the exact distance will not work. Lee, and other researchers following him, have looked at other activities, e.g., cricket bowlers running up to the bowling crease, and found the same results.

The most dramatic examples of the control of movement caused by perception–action coupling, however, were probably those found in games like table tennis. Bootsma and Van Wieringen (1990) have shown that as table tennis players move to hit a ball, they are constantly altering the position of their bat and arm with reference to their position in relation to the ball. Of particular interest in this study was the nature of the movements made by the arm. Bootsma and Van Wieringen used the term *funnel shape* to explain this. It does not mean that the bat followed a funnel shape but that the initial stages of the movement were rather general and became more precise as they approached the point of contact. Small alterations were made to the direction of movement to ensure the best point of contact. Moreover, movement was altered with regard to momentum so that the bat was accelerating at the time of contact. In Chapter 2, we also talked about the way in which τ controlled the direction and speed of movement when moving to catch a ball. In all of these cases the movement is under joint perception–action control, which is dealt with at peripheral level, with little or no recourse to the CNS.

Discussion

In this section, I will summarize how Information Processing Theory and the ecological psychology theories, Action Systems and Dynamical Systems, explain movement control. Following that we will examine some of the strengths and weaknesses of the two perspectives.

Due to criticisms by ecological psychologists and questions asked by Information Processing theorists themselves, the way in which Information Processing Theory accounts for motor control has been altered fairly dramatically in recent years. Nevertheless, efferent organization taking place in the motor cortex is still thought to be the most important factor. Most Information Processing theorists believe that what is organized is instructions regarding the movement rather than commands to specific muscles. Fine tuning of these CNS commands is thought to be undertaken by the lower centres of the CNS, the basal ganglia and cerebellum, and by $\alpha-\gamma$ co-activation in the PNS. It is believed that feedforward, from the motor cortex, provides these areas with the necessary information to undertake changes. The extent that such changes can be made is limited, however. Movements of less than one reaction time are thought to be under open-loop control, although feedforward to the basal ganglia and muscle spindles can ensure that there is no mismatch between the intended outcome and the actual outcome. Movements greater than one reaction time are under closed-loop control. They are affected by feedback from the PNS, with the cerebellum playing a key role in their control. The sensory and motor cortices are seen as the main controllers of such movement. Automatic well-learnt movements are believed to form motor programs, which are performed in an open-loop manner.

To the ecological psychologists, the role of the motor cortex is to issue very general commands. These are in no way specific and do not represent instructions to the limbs. The movement of the limbs is controlled by the interaction between the environment, the task and the individual. Each environment, task and person brings certain constraints that affect the way in which the movement is carried out. The body is believed to be self-organizing and, although feedback to the cerebellum may help control movement, it is claimed that more basic interactions between muscles, joints and the environment control most of the movement. Control is ongoing and is an interaction between perception and action. Even visual proprioception takes place at a peripheral level, without recourse to the CNS. Table 7.1 provides an outline of the basics of how each theory explains motor control.

One of the major criticisms of Information Processing Theory, with regard to motor control, has been its inability to provide an adequate explanation for the control of movements of less than one reaction time. The idea of an open-loop operation, with no recourse to feedback once an action has begun, looked very appealing in the 1970s. Minor alterations of movements, in less than one reaction time, were accounted for by feedforward. However, research such as that by Bootsma and Van Wieringen raised questions for which Information Processing Theory has failed to provide a fully satisfactory explanation.

Table 7.1 Ecological psychology and Information Processing Theory explanations of motor control

	Information Processing Theory	Dynamical Systems Theory
Central Nervous System	1. Selects movement commands 2. Feeds forward to basal ganglia and cerebellum 3. Holds outcome in memory	1. Selects general goals
Peripheral Nervous System	1. Spinal cord: (a) relays information to the muscles; (b) has some control via feedforward ($\alpha-\gamma$ co-activation); (c) relays information back to cerebellum and sensory cortex	1. Organizes movement – choice of limbs 2. Limbs are self-organizing 3. Becomes attuned to affordances

The second major criticism of Information Processing Theory explanations of motor control is based on the problem of storing a huge amount of specific motor programs. Schmidt tried to explain this by saying that we store schemas, not specific motor programs. The schemas form generalized motor programs, which can be altered for each particular situation. Again this has satisfied many psychologists but by no means all. It is still thought, by many, that this is too simplistic an answer, given the considerable number of movements that humans, and indeed other animals, can make.

The major criticism of ecological psychology explanations is a failure to account for how we improve with practice. If all necessary information is in the environment and action is self-organizing, based on natural laws, surely we would be able to perform the skill the first time without any problem. Learning would not be necessary. The ecological psychologists argue that with practice we become more attuned to what the environment affords and self-organization of movement becomes more efficient. So far, they have not provided very satisfactory explanations of how this occurs.

To many, the use of τ to explain the perception–action interaction in interceptive actions and in moving to a target is one of the strongest points in favour of an ecological approach to motor control. To others, it is totally the opposite. It is difficult, for many psychologists, to accept that τ simply triggers off a movement without recourse to some CNS activity. The idea that we are born with an innate capacity to know when to move in order to intercept appears inconceivable to many.

The biggest difficulty for ecological psychologists, however, would appear to be their failure to explain why comparatively large changes in movement cannot be made in less than one reaction time. As we saw in the Bootsma and Van Wieringen studies the changes in movement are small. McLeod (1987), examining cricket, showed that if the alterations needed were comparatively large the person could not make the necessary changes until after one reaction time. McGarry and Franks (1997), in a series of experiments, have shown that if you ask a person to move a rod in one direction and then reverse the movement on a given signal, they cannot do so in less than one reaction time.

So you can see that, although both theories have some good explanations of motor control, neither is perfect. Information Processing theorists have been forced to change many of their original ideas based on the evidence of modern techniques of observation. At first there might appear to be reluctance on the part of the ecological psychologists to accept that the CNS may play a more important role than they so far advocate. However, ecological psychologists are quick to point out that they have never denied that the CNS plays a part in motor control. They claim that we cannot, at this moment in time, know exactly what the CNS does, due to limitations in measurement of CNS activity. Therefore, they will continue to try to explain motor control, as best they can, without recourse to the CNS. More recently, it has been advocated that a hybrid explanation, combining both theories, may be the best method of explaining movement.

Key points

Information Processing Theory and motor control

- Proprioception is the ability of the person to know where their body is in space and to be aware of the position of different limbs.

- Visual proprioception is the use of vision to aid movement:

  - it is primarily the role of ambient vision.

- Vestibular apparatus provides information concerning:

  - balance,

- o direction of movement.

- The PNS carries neural messages from and to the CNS, and this occurs in the spinal cord:

  - o efferent or motor (motoneurons) nerves take messages from the CNS to the limbs,

  - o afferent or sensory nerves take information from the senses to the CNS,

  - o movement can be controlled to some extent in the spinal cord by $\alpha-\gamma$ co-activation (allows alterations to be made in less than one reaction time).

- The CNS organizes movement:

  - o instructions are sent by the motor cortex to the basal ganglia, cerebellum and spinal cord.

- Movements of less than one reaction time are controlled by the basal ganglia:

  - o feedforward from the motor cortex allows it to make minor alterations where necessary.

- Movements of greater than one reaction time are controlled by the cerebellum:

  - o the cerebellum receives feedback from the spinal cord, thus allowing it to alter movements if necessary.

- Well-learned movements become automatic and are said to have developed into motor programs:

  - o motor programs can be performed without recourse to feedback,

  - o according to Schema Theory, motor programs are generalized, i.e., they can be adapted to suit different conditions.

Ecological psychology and motor control

- The CNS decides what movement to make:

  - instructions from the CNS are functionally specific (they merely outline what needs to be done, there is no detail).

- Movement is controlled by the PNS:

  - muscles, tendons and nerves interact to control the movement – they are self-organized.

- Self-organization is dependent on task, environmental and organismic constraints:

  - task constraints are factors such as rules of a competition (e.g., there can only be a one footed take off in the high jump) or the laws of science affecting the best way to do something (e.g., a long lever is necessary in the discus, if it is to be thrown a long way),

  - environmental constraints are determined by the situation in which the skill must be performed (e.g., running on sand demands different self-organization to running on a tartan track),

  - organismic constraints are the person's physical, mental and emotional qualities,

  - different organismic constraints mean that self-organization for doing the same task will differ between two people (e.g., Maurice Greene and Michael Johnson sprinting).

- Self-organization allows us to control the degrees of freedom (all the muscles, joints, nerves, etc. that are involved in any movement).

- Visual guidance of movement is controlled by τ (time to contact).

Test your knowledge

(Answers in Appendix 3.)

Part one

Below are a number of questions (Q) and answers (A). Fill in the spaces using the phrases below.

1. Q. How did Sherrington (1906) describe _____ ?

    A. The perception of the body and its position in space.

2. Q. What does the term _____ describe?

    A. The person's perception of the movements of their body and separate body parts.

3. Q. What are the two types of _____ ?

    A. Horizontal and vertical.

4. Q. To what does the _____ refer?

    A. The interaction between the oculomotor system and the vestibular apparatus.

5. Q. Which part of the vestibular apparatus is responsible for the perception of the _____ and changes in acceleration?

    A. Semi-circular canals.

6. Q. Which afferent nerves are situated _____ ?

    A. Golgi tendon organs.

7. Q. Which part of the CNS initiates _____ ?

A. Pre-motor cortex.

8. Q. Which part of the brain is thought to regulate movements of _____?

A. Basal ganglia.

9. Q. What is the name given to the process also known as _____?

A. $\alpha-\gamma$ co-activation.

10. Q. Which part of the brain controls _____?

A. The cerebellum.

11. Q. Which nerves are responsible for passing information from the CNS to the muscles so that _____?

A. Motoneurons or efferent nerves.

12. Q. Which nerves are responsible for passing information _____ to the CNS?

A. Sensory or afferent nerves.

13. Q. What did Keele (1968) describe as a _____ that allows movement to be performed without any peripheral feedback?

A. A motor program.

14. Q. What do Information Processing theorists call the process which allows us to make _____ to movements in less than one reaction time?

A. Feedforward.

15. Q. According to ecological psychologists, what is the _____?

A. To set the goal.

16. Q. What do ecological psychologists mean by _____?

   A. The physical and mental characteristics of the individual, which affect the way in which they carry out a movement.

17. Q. What kind of constraints are _____?

   A. Task constraints.

18. Q. How do ecological psychologists describe different _____?

   A. Self-organization.

19. Q. What term did Bernstein (1967) use to describe the number of _____ that must be controlled in order to produce a co-ordinated movement?

   A. Degrees of freedom.

20. Q. What name did Lee and Young (1985) give to the time when information from an object results in _____?

   A. τ.

Vestibulo–oculomotor interaction
movement can take place
between muscles and joints
less than one reaction time
muscles, joints and nerves
voluntary movement
about a movement
muscles and joints working together
initiation of a movement to intercept
movements of greater than one reaction time

set of muscle commands
direction of movement
short-loop feedback
minor alterations
long-loop feedback
organismic constraints

rules of a game
role of the CNS
kinesthesis
proprioception
peripheral vision

Part two

Fill in the blank spaces using words taken from the list below (NB there are more words in the list than there are spaces).

1. There are two types of peripheral vision, _____ and _____.

2. _____ is the most important of the senses with regard to proprioception.

3. We visually track fast movements using _____.

4. The _____ and _____ provide information about the position of the head.

5. The _____ motoneurons inform the muscle spindles about the tension they should 'feel'.

6. Movements of more than one reaction time are said to be under _____ loop control.

7. According to Keele (1968), when developing a motor program we firstly form a _____ of the task.

8. Keele (1968) claimed that the development of motor programs takes place in the motor cortex, basal ganglia and _____.

9. An Arab spring, flick-flack and somersault, performed as a gymnastics routine, is an example of an _____ motor program.

10. MacNeilage (1980) believed that we store the _____ of key points in a movement.

11. Schmidt (1975) claimed that we do not store specifics of a motor program but _____ rules or schemas.

12. Schmidt's theory explains how we can do the same skill in a _____ of different ways.

13. Sherrington (1906) asked whether CNS instructions were _____ or _____ commands.

14. According to ecological psychologists, commands from the CNS are _____ _____.

15. Two people will perform the same skill differently because they have different _____ constraints.

16. A baseball pitcher and a cricket bowler use different actions because of the _____ constraints under which they must perform.

17. Someone doing a somersault in a gymnasium on a sprung floor and then doing the same action on grass will need to alter their movement because of the differing _____ constraints.

18. According to ecological psychologists, we do not need to remember a movement because our limbs will carry it out automatically because of _____.

19. According to Lee and Young (1985), action and perception of the τ margin occur _____.

20. Bootsma and Van Wieringen (1990) used the term _____ shape to explain how we control late movement of a bat when striking a ball.

utricles	funnel	distance	task	location	short
functionally	template	saccades	muscle	ambient	gamma
cerebellum	long	organismic	alpha	generalized	movement
specific	vision	horizontal	executive	automatically	
peripheral	variety	environmental	saccules	self-organization	

Additional reading

Sugden D (2002) Moving forward to dynamic choices: David Sugden, University of Leeds, PEAUK Fellow Lecture, 4 December 2001. *Brit J Teaching Phys Educ* **33**: 6–8; 25

Wrisberg CA (2000) Movement production and motor programs. In: *Study guide for motor learning and performance*, Wrisberg CA (Ed) Human Kinetics, Champaign, Illinois, USA, pp. 53–66

8 Learning

Learning Objectives

By the end of this chapter, you should be able to

♦ define learning

♦ understand how we measure 'learning'

♦ understand the nature of explicit and implicit learning

♦ understand the nature and role of instruction

♦ understand the nature and role of demonstrations

♦ understand selected cognitive theories of learning

  ◊ Fitts and Posner's theory

  ◊ Gentile's theory

  ◊ Adams' theory

  ◊ Schmidt's Schema Theory

  ◊ Observational Learning Theory

♦ understand how Dynamical Systems Theory explains learning

♦ understand how developmental factors affect learning

  ◊ cognitive development

  ◊ motor development

♦ understand the practical implications for coaches and performers

Acquisition and Performance of Sports Skills   T. McMorris
© 2004 John Wiley & Sons, Ltd   ISBNs: 0-470-84994-0 (HB); 0-470-84995-9 (PB)

Introduction

We often hear coaches say, 'he/she is learning'. They normally say this after the athlete has had a good performance following a number of poor displays. Everyone knows that the coach means that, although the player did well today, he/she has not fully learnt yet. In fact, they are talking about the difference between learning and performance. Kerr defined *performance* as being '*a temporary occurrence fluctuating from time to time: something which is transitory*' (Kerr, 1982). We are not thought to have fully learnt a skill until we can perform it with some *consistency*. The process of acquiring this consistency is what we mean by learning; '*learning is a relatively permanent change in performance resulting from practice or past experience*' (Kerr, 1982).

The term 'relatively permanent' means the same as being consistent. It is a more accurate description because no one can be totally consistent, as there are many, many factors that affect performance, of which learning is only one. Even when a skill is automatic we find ourselves underachieving from time to time. Tiger Woods actually misses simple putts, but not very often. I also miss simple putts. Unlike Tiger Woods, I have played very little golf, therefore there is some doubt as to whether I am capable of making these shots. We know that Woods is capable. Woods' *capability* to make the putt represents his learning. My non-capability means that I have not learnt yet. Judging by my last attempts, I probably never will.

Measuring learning

The fact that performance fluctuates, even for very skilful performers, leads to a problem in how we measure learning. At this moment in time, *we can only measure learning by observing performance*. Figure 8.1 shows the performance of one of my students throwing 10 darts, with her non-preferred hand, at a concentric target. The centre circle scored 10 points, the next nine and so on. It is not surprising that her scores fluctuate greatly. Figure 8.2 shows her mean performance following 10, 20, 30, 40, 50 and 60 practice trials, respectively. As you can see, her mean scores show an improvement from her first 10 trials, but after 40 trials she performed worse than after 30 trials. This was mostly due to two very poor throws. Overall she showed signs of improving, as can be seen by the dotted line. After 60 trials she scored a comparatively high mean and was more consistent than in the other trials. Her results, however, cannot say what would have happened if we tested her in another set of trials. Nor do they

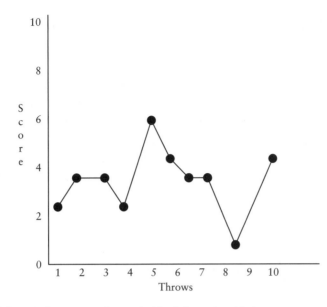

Figure 8.1 Performance of an individual throwing 10 darts at a concentric target

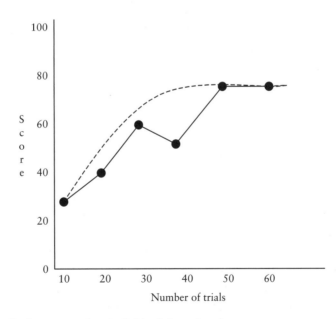

Figure 8.2 Performance of an individual throwing darts at a target, over a series of trials

say anything about consistency. We need better measures than these to examine learning. Strictly speaking *we cannot actually measure learning*, we can only *infer it based on performance*.

The three most commonly used methods for inferring learning are the use of *retention tests*, transfer tests and the plotting of performance curves. Retention, you will remember, is the persistence of performance over a period of no practice. As such, it should measure consistency and capability. The example, above, of the student learning to throw darts with her non-preferred hand demonstrates only performance, it does not examine retention. In order to examine her ability to retain the performance, we would have to re-test her again after a period of no learning. We could then decide how much she had retained and, therefore, how much she had learnt. The major problem with such tests is deciding how long a period of no practice we have. If we have too great a time, forgetting will occur due to decay. However, if we have too short a period, we may well only be continuing our measure of performance again rather than retention. This is a major problem for researchers in this field. Some researchers use a second retention test, called a post-retention test, in order to examine retention over more than one time period.

The use of *transfer tasks*, to infer learning, is based on the assumption that if a skill is truly learnt it can be performed in a number of different environments or situations. A method of transfer might be changing the task demands, e.g., learning to pass a basketball unopposed and then having to pass it while someone tries to intercept the pass. Another method is by changing the environment, e.g., moving from playing short tennis (tennis on a modified small court) to playing on a full-size court.

Measuring learning by *performance curves* is similar to our example of the student throwing darts. Performance of the learner is plotted over a period of time and/or a number of trials and is shown graphically. Figure 8.3(a) shows the curve for a student performing a basketball set shot. He threw 10 sets of 10 trials. His mean score for each set of 10 was plotted and then depicted graphically. The curve was smoothed out to show a typical performance curve. It should be noted that performance curves are sometimes inaccurately called learning curves. This was the norm in the early literature.

There are four common types of curve that have been found by researchers. Our basketball player demonstrated a *positively accelerated curve*. There is an overall general improvement, as we can see it is slow at first and then accelerates. Figure 8.3(b) shows a *negatively accelerated curve*. There is an early improvement but then performance tapers off somewhat. Figure 8.3(c) shows a *linear* improvement with practice. While Figure 8.3(d) demonstrates an *ogive* or *S-shaped curve*.

The curve in Figure 8.4 demonstrates the effect of what we call a *plateau* in learning. This is quite a common occurrence in learning and is probably something you have experienced yourself. There comes a point when practising does not appear to be having any effect, this is the plateau. If we keep on

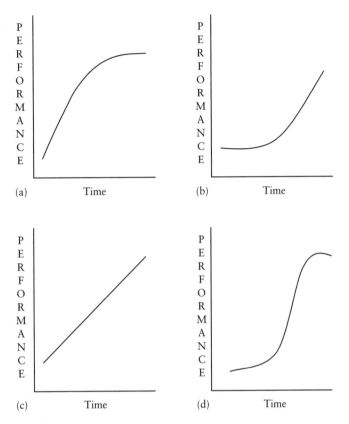

Figure 8.3 Examples of typical performance curves

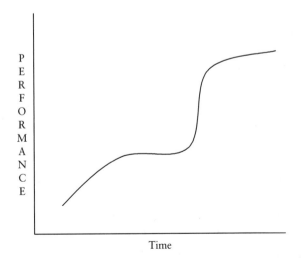

Figure 8.4 Example of a performance curve showing a plateauing effect

practising, there is a break through and more learning is demonstrated. Of course, sometimes what appears to be a plateau is in effect the limit of our capability and no more improvement is demonstrated, regardless of the amount of practice we undertake.

There are a number of reasons why plateaus might occur. It is possible that boredom, or reactive inhibition, is causing a temporary hold on performance. To the Information Processing theorists, however, a more likely explanation comes from the nature of memory. As you will recall from Chapter 6, it takes time for engrams in the memory to be formed and this is what may be happening when a plateau is observed. It may also be that, in fact, there is no such thing as a plateau and that the problem is in the limitations of measuring performance. Evidence from studies using kinematic assessment shows that there are changes in the way in which the skill is being performed, which do not produce an immediate quantitative change in performance but which do so over time.

Another problem facing the researcher into learning is the choice of what task to use to measure learning. Very little research has examined tasks that we would consider to be *ecologically valid* with regard to sports performance. Most tasks have been laboratory-based skills and mostly fine motor rather than gross body skills. Indeed, a great deal of what we read about learning motor skills is based on research into learning verbal skills. There are two basic reasons for this. The first is that if we use ecologically valid skills, e.g., hitting a golf ball, our research is going to be affected by the participants' previous experience. If they are all at different levels of capability, at the beginning of the experiment, it is very difficult to determine how much learning has taken place. It is also difficult to control for what researchers call *intervening variables*, e.g., environmental factors which will affect the task.

Geert Savelsbergh, one of the leading ecological psychology researchers, while giving a presentation at University College Chichester, criticized his own research into τ as lacking ecological validity. He had participants catching a ball, while in a sitting position and when the ball trajectory was known. Savelsbergh had to compromise between being truly ecologically valid and being able to control his experiment. The task used by Savelsbergh, however, was more ecologically valid than some of the tasks used by Information Processing researchers. They use skills like *mirror tracing* and *placing pegs into a pegboard*. In mirror tracing, the person must trace a figure while they can only see their hand in a mirror. In the pegboard task, they have to place the pegs into the board as quickly as possible. It is often done with the non-preferred hand. Such experiments are not affected by past experience but may have little transfer to real-life skills. In recent times, more ecologically valid experiments have been undertaken but we still need far more before we can be 100 per cent confident about the findings.

So far in this section, we have assumed that learning is always *positive*, i.e., through experience we improve. This is not necessarily the case. Leaning can be *negative*. We can develop inappropriate responses. We may, also, change from performing a skill properly to performing it badly.

In the next two sections of this chapter, we will examine how Information Processing theorists account for learning and look at some of the research that supports their claims. In the section following that, we will examine the case put by the ecological psychologists.

Information Processing Theory and learning

To the Information Processing theorists, motor learning is about increasing one's LTMM store – in particular, developing motor programs. Learning movements is primarily a CNS task. This does not mean, however, that the PNS is not affected by learning. Learning is represented in the CNS by the development of neural interconnections. Similarly, it is thought that the pathways from the CNS to the muscles become more streamlined as we learn. In other words, the neural interconnections in the PNS become stronger. This is shown by an improvement in co-ordination and can be observed by the fact that the learner appears to be performing more easily and in a smoother manner than the beginner. I think of the development of these neural pathways as being similar to when we walk across a field of high grass. At first, it is difficult and there is no clear pathway. After time, however, we wear down the grass in certain areas to produce a clear pathway across the field. This is what is happening in the PNS.

This cognitive, CNS dominated, idea of learning led Anderson to develop his ACT Theory. We have already touched on this briefly in Chapter 3. Anderson believes that the first stage of learning is to acquire *declarative knowledge*. Declarative knowledge is *knowing what to do*. When we listen to instructions or watch someone performing a skill, we work out how to do it. Thus, we are developing declarative knowledge. As we practice, we move from possessing declarative knowledge to possessing *procedural knowledge*. Procedural knowledge means *being able to do the skill*. Although Anderson's theory was developed for verbal skills, it has had a large following in the motor learning field. As we stated in Chapter 3, there is no proof that we move from declarative to procedural knowledge. Indeed, recent research examining implicit learning suggests strongly that we can obtain procedural knowledge without ever having declarative knowledge of the skill (Masters, 2000).

It was thought, until very recently, that we could only acquire skills if we consciously set out to learn them. Richard Magill and associates (see Magill, 1993), however, showed that we could learn at a sub-conscious level, what has become termed as *implicit learning*. Following Magill's research, Richard Masters (see Masters, 2000) has carried out a great deal of research into implicit learning, most of it being ecologically valid. He has shown that exposure to a skill, even when one is not consciously paying attention to it, can result in learning of at least as good value as when we have learnt explicitly. *Explicit learning* refers to what we might call the 'normal' way of learning. We are given overt, or explicit, instructions and told to concentrate on the task at hand.

I am sure that you have all experienced implicit learning in some way or other. We very often learn pop songs this way. I bet that nearly all of you have found yourselves singing a song and thinking, 'Why am I singing *that* song? – I *hate* it'. I first came across implicit learning many years before I had heard of it as a psychological phenomenon. I played cricket for a team whose ground was next to a fun-fair. Although I never paid any attention to the noises coming from the fun-fair, every Sunday, following Saturday's game, I could repeat the songs that had been played on the fun-fair loudspeaker system (some cruel people claimed that I could only recall the words and that the tunes were unrecognizable).

Although the phenomenon of implicit learning is now accepted by Information Processing theorists, it is difficult to reconcile with the theory. Obviously Information Processing theorists need to revise, to some extent, the notion of perceptual filters which we covered in Chapter 1 when looking at selective attention. It would appear that even stimuli, which we do not overtly rehearse, can pass into LTM.

While implicit learning may be difficult for Information Processing theorists to explain, another phenomenon – the effect of *mental rehearsal* – supports the notion of CNS control of movement. It has been known for many years that mentally rehearsing skills aids learning and performance. Most researchers, however, claim that mental rehearsal only works *in conjunction with physical rehearsal*. Research has shown that individuals who use mental rehearsal, as well as physical rehearsal, do learn more quickly than those using physical rehearsal only. One theory put forward to explain the advantages of mental rehearsal is that by thinking about the skill we build up a picture or model, in the CNS, of how the skill should be performed. This is similar to Anderson's idea of developing declarative knowledge, which in turn is not dissimilar to

Keele's notion of acquiring a motor program by developing a template of the skill.

The second theory concerning how mental rehearsal works is based on the idea that the CNS cannot differentiate between mental activity, in its own right, and mental activity that leads to motor performance. Thus, *if we think about doing something the CNS learns the same, or almost the same, as actually doing the task*. Hale (1982) provided some experimental support for this. He had people mentally rehearse doing a task. While they were rehearsing, he had EMGs fitted to the muscles that would be used if they were actually doing the skill. He showed that there was some neural activity even though they never overtly moved.

There are different kinds of mental rehearsal. Some people simply think through how to do the task, using verbal self-instructions. The most common form of mental rehearsal, however, is through *mental imagery*. In mental imagery the person sees themselves doing the skill. It is believed that, in this way, they experience the task almost as well as if they were actually doing it. Mental imagery is better known as a tool used by sports psychologists in trying to help athletes overcome anxiety. It has become forgotten that it can also aid learning. It is especially useful if the performer is injured and so cannot practice.

Instruction

To the Information Processing theorists, instruction is vital because they believe that learning is dependent on CNS activity. We need to be told or see what to do. This does not have to be done explicitly or overtly. As we have seen, we can learn implicitly. In learning implicitly, however, we still have to see or hear what it is to be learnt.

In the early years of the development of motor learning as an academic study, a fair amount of research was carried out into instruction. In recent years, however, little has been undertaken. The most commonly researched area has been to compare *verbal, visual and verbal plus visual* instruction. Based on the 'a picture paints a thousand words' idea, most researchers have hypothesized that visual instruction will be better than verbal. In general this has been found to be the case but not unequivocally. We would expect visual instruction to be superior to verbal because it is not possible to verbally articulate many skills. Try it: choose a skill from your own favourite sport and try to write down an explanation of how to perform it.

It is, however, possible to verbally articulate some skills. Moreover, the notion that a demonstration is easy to follow is something of an exaggeration. In teaching the triple jump, for example, I found that the perception of what had been demonstrated varied from child to child. Yet they saw exactly the same demonstration. Very often when we use visual instruction, or demonstration, we assume that the learner is paying attention to the key points. This may well not be the case. It is, therefore, no surprise that the most successful method of instruction is verbal plus visual. In this, the learner can see the movement and the instructor can verbally point out what the person should look for.

One area of research which has received little attention is that of the interaction between the type of skill and the type of instruction. One my former students, Paul Britton, carried out a study where he used verbal or visual instruction with a discrete skill, the basketball set shot, and a serial skill, the lay-up. He found that verbal instruction was as good as visual for the set shot but not for the lay-up. This is related to the problem of verbal articulation. It was comparatively easy for the children to understand the verbal instructions for the less complex set shot than for the lay-up.

There would appear to be little doubt that, where possible, we should use verbal plus visual instruction. However, this is not always possible. In Britain, at the moment, it is recommended, for safety reasons, to teach swimming from the poolside. Also, we may simply not be able to do the skill ourselves. If this is the case, we must work hard at making sure that the verbal instructions are easily understandable to the learner. We cannot use jargon, if the learners do not understand it. In my first year of teaching I observed a colleague teaching soccer to a group of 11-year old boys. One of the boys had the ball and just stood still, obviously not knowing what to do. The teacher shouted, 'carry it' – soccer jargon for run with the ball at your feet. The boy immediately bent down, picked the ball up and ran forward. When the teacher shouted at him for being foolish, he was totally bemused. Not only is jargon to be avoided but we must also be careful about the words we use. Although we may not think of ourselves as having a large vocabulary we have, compared with many people, especially children. Therefore, we should use words that we are sure the person understands. In Chapter 6, we looked at the limitations of STM and we should take that into account. Keep what we have to say down to a minimum. There is a danger with coaches and teachers that they think they have to be constantly making comments and giving instructions, this is not so.

Demonstration

In the above section, we talked about visual instruction which of course is also known as demonstration. In this section, I will not repeat what was said above.

Instead, we will concentrate on some of the key issues concerning the quality of demonstration and its motivational aspects. If we want people to learn by observation, the demonstration needs to be correct. If the demonstration is incorrect, there is every chance of the person copying the incorrect movement. This means that there will be some skills that the coach or teacher cannot demonstrate, because their own performance level is not good enough. However, there has to be some kind of compromise. The instructor needs to decide whether his/her level of performance is satisfactory to demonstrate the skill. The demonstration needs to be adequate, not perfect. Some people overcome limitations by demonstrating in slow motion. I have major problems with this. If you are to use this method, you must make sure that speed is not an essential factor in the performance of the skill. In watching coaches demonstrate dribbling in soccer, using the slow-motion method, I regularly observe the fact that the learners fail to accelerate when going past their opponent. This is almost certainly because the slow-motion demonstration does not show this aspect of the skill. Yet it is a vital part of the skill.

Slow-motion demonstrations may, however, be necessary in some cases even when the instructor can demonstrate at normal speed. Some skills are performed too quickly for the learner to see exactly what is happening. Throwing combination punches in boxing can happen too quickly for the beginner to perceive properly. In such cases the instructor will have to give a slow-motion demonstration. However, I would argue very strongly that this should be done only after a real-time demonstration has been carried out. The same applies for learning dance routines.

As well as being instructional, demonstration can also be motivational. The learner should observe the demonstration and think, 'I want to do that'. However, they must also think, 'I can do that'. This latter point highlights a problem with coaches and teachers demonstrating skills, especially to children. The child must perceive that children can also perform this skill, it is not something that only adults can do. This has led researchers to examine the use of peer demonstrations. Instead of the instructor giving the demonstration themselves, they get someone of the same age as the learners to perform the skill. This may be done directly or on a film, if there is no one in the group who can perform the skill. In one class, to which I taught swimming, I often used one of the boys, who was a good swimmer, to demonstrate the different strokes. This, also, overcame the fact that I was not allowed get into the pool with them. Peer demonstration can also be used if you feel the instructor knows that someone in the group can perform the skill better than they themselves. On one FA Coaching course that I taught, I had the former Bristol City player Alan Walsh as one of the trainee coaches. Alan had one of the hardest shots in football. Therefore, when we examined shooting it was obviously more sensible to let him demonstrate rather than do it myself.

Although I have been talking about the problems of learners being so overawed by demonstrations that they feel they cannot achieve success, it is sometimes best to show a film of a top-class athlete performing a skill. This can have great motivational value. When Torvill and Dean were at the height of their success in ice dance many aspiring ice dancers tried to copy what they did. Similarly, Australia is full of Brett Lee 'wannabees' all trying to bowl a fast outswinger. This kind of demonstration is probably best used with athletes who are past the initial stages of learning, but it can be very motivational. One of the most startling examples of how performance by an expert can act as a motivational tool came following the 1974 soccer World Cup Final. In that game the Dutch star Johann Cruyff first performed what has become known as the 'Cruyff turn'. Despite the fact that this way of turning had never been seen before, by the beginning of the next English soccer season players in every standard from the First Division (now the Premiership) to local parks players were using the 'Cruyff turn'. This was only 6 weeks later.

Cognitivist theories of learning

The earliest theories of learning were developed by the behaviourists. They were based on animal studies and were concerned with the development of a relationship between a stimulus and a response, hence they were often called *stimulus–response (S–R) Bond* theories. One of the best known S–R Bond theorists was Skinner. Skinner experimented with pigeons and showed that, by rewarding a pigeon with food every time it pressed a lever with its beak, he could get the pigeon to press the lever whenever it was available. So the stimulus was the lever and the pressing the response. Based on such studies, the behaviourists argued that humans worked in the same way and built up a vast amount of S–R Bonds.

The early cognitivists, e.g., the Gestältists, felt that this was too simplistic for humans. The Gestältists believed that humans perceive a problem and try to determine, logically, what the best possible answer to the problem is. They might engage in actual physical trial and error as well as thinking through the problem. Eventually they would find a solution. They called this the *'eureka' moment*, after the word used by the Greek philosopher Archimedes on discovering the principle of density. Despite the intervention of the Gestältists, S–R Bond theories remained popular until Information Processing Theory gained the ascendancy among psychologists. There are numerous Information

Processing based theories of learning. I will not attempt to even name them all, never mind explain them all. In the following sections we will simply outline the most prominent of these theories.

Fitts and Posner's Three Stage Theory

The first theory to be widely held, and indeed it is still considered valid today, was put forward by Paul Fitts and Michael Posner (1967). Fitts and Posner claimed that learning took place in three stages: the cognitive, associative and autonomous. In the *cognitive* stage the person tries to make sense of instructions. They make a great deal of use of verbal labels. This does not mean that instruction needs to be verbal, but simply that the individual uses verbalization to aid memory. The length of this period will depend on the nature of the task. In skills requiring perception and decision making, there are often mistakes made and the person attends to irrelevant as well as relevant stimuli. The motor component is characterized by crude unco-ordinated movement.

With practice the individual develops the knowledge of what to do (very similar to Anderson's declarative knowledge stage). When someone is at this stage they are said to be in the *associative* stage (sometimes called the intermediate stage). At this stage, practice is required to perfect the skill and develop the consistent co-ordinative movement that demonstrates learning. When the person can perform consistently and with little overt cognitive activity, they are said to have reached the *autonomous* stage. Although performance at this stage is rarely affected by distraction and stress, it is difficult to alter. This can be negative if the person has developed responses, or aspects of the response, which are inappropriate.

Gentile's Model of Learning

While Fitts and Posner's theory is basically a general cognitive theory, Gentile (1972) follows very much an Information Processing model. Gentile divides learning into two stages, but there are eight steps to stage one. Stage one is called the *initial skill acquisition stage*. You can see the steps which make up this stage in Table 8.1. Here I will try to précis Gentile's explanation of the stage. The first aim is to get an idea of what the movement involves. The learner must then learn to differentiate between relevant and irrelevant cues. Thus, selective attention is developed. The person then formulates an action plan, i.e., what to do. This is very similar to Fitts and Posner's cognitive stage.

Table 8.1 Steps in Gentile *et al.*'s initial skill acquisition stage of learning (based on Gentile *et al.*, 1975)

Step	
1	Goal-directed behaviour activated
2	Population of stimuli established
3	Selective attention developed
4	Motor-plan formulated
5	Plan of action initiated
6	Actual movement compared to goal and action plan
7	KR and KP used to modify plan
8	Act

The next steps in Gentile's initial skill acquisition phase are similar to Fitts and Posner's associative stage. The individual uses feedback to correct inappropriate responses and to reinforce correct movements. Thus, we can see that this stage, as a whole, is very much dependent on the development of a LTM store. Perception–decision–efferent organization and feedback are seen as the key factors. There could be said to be little that is different to Keele's idea of how motor programs are developed. The final part of Gentile's model is called the *skill refinement* stage. It is characterized by what Gentile called *fixation and diversification*. She describes these processes as being the refinement of closed skills and the ability to use the movement in open-skill situations. This is, of course, similar to developing a specific motor program into a more generalized one.

Adams' Closed-loop Theory of Learning

Although Adams (1971) developed his theory slightly ahead of Gentile, I have chosen to deal with Adams after Gentile because his theory leads into that of Schmidt, which we will examine next. Adams was unhappy with the open-loop motor program idea of motor control. Observation of movements show that we constantly monitor movement as it is taking place, especially movements of more than one reaction time. In other words, he saw movement as being a closed-loop operation. Adams, therefore, set out to explain how we acquire the ability to do this. He believed that, as we learn a skill, we develop what he called the *perceptual* trace. The perceptual trace is memory for the feel of successful past movements. Once we have developed the perceptual trace, we can compare the trace with the feel of the ongoing movement. This allows us to correct inappropriate actions. An essential part of developing the perceptual trace is that we need to know how accurate or successful our responses were. The more successful, the stronger the trace will become.

Adams was aware that the role of the perceptual trace was to control an already ongoing movement. The movement would have to be initiated by some other control mechanism. This he called the *memory trace*. According to Adams, the memory trace was responsible for the selection and initiation of the movement. This is not dissimilar to the joint open–closed loop control of movement that we commented on in the previous chapter.

Adams believed that the development of the perceptual and memory traces was achieved in two stages. The first stage he called the *verbal–motor stage*. This stage is really a combination of Fitts and Posner's verbal and associative stages. Adams' final stage, the *motor stage*, is similar to Fitts and Posner's autonomous stage. In this stage, Adams believes that the individual strengthens the perceptual and memory traces until they can be used automatically, thus taking up little CNS channel space.

Schmidt's Schema Theory

Like all good scientists, Jack Adams was not fully satisfied with his theory and he encouraged his students not only to question it but to try to come up with answers that would deal with its weaknesses. One of Adams' students, Richard Schmidt, identified two major problems with Adams' theory. First of all, although there is an open-loop element to it, this only applies to the early part of a movement. The theory does not explain how we make fast movements of less than one reaction time. Schmidt could of course point to Keele's motor program theory to explain this. However, Schmidt was aware of the specificity problem in motor-program theory. No cognitivists could explain how we are able to perform novel skills or a large number of variations of the same skill. This is what Schema Theory (Schmidt, 1975) set out to do (Figure 8.5).

We have touched briefly on the notion of what a schema is in Chapter 7. Schmidt believes that we do not develop specific motor programs but schemas. A schema is a set of generalized rules or rules which are generic to a group of movements. Like Adams, Schmidt believed that memory for movement was of two kinds, these he called the recall and recognition memories. Like Adams' memory trace, the *recall memory* is responsible for the choice and initiation of action. While the *recognition memory* evaluates the ongoing movement and makes appropriate changes in the action. This is the role Adams described as

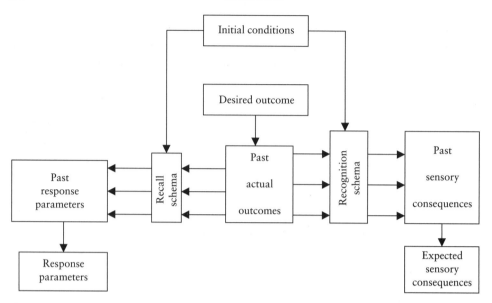

Figure 8.5 Model of Schema Theory (adapted from Schmidt, 1975); reproduced with permission of the American Psychological Association from Psych. Rev **82**: 225–260

being undertaken by the perceptual trace. The major difference, however, is that Adams believed that the traces were memories of specific movements, whereas Schmidt argued that they were generalized.

Schmidt states that the learning of the recall and recognition schemas are brought about by the development of the general rules which we develop during performance. In developing the recall schema, we remember *the desired outcome, the initial conditions, the response parameters and the sensory consequences*. An example of initial conditions would be the position of the individual's body parts when preparing to play a forehand drive in tennis. The speed, line and length of ball flight would also be initial conditions. Response parameters, sometimes called *response specifications*, are changes in the specifics of the action which are necessary if we are to be successful.

These parameters will depend on the situation in which we find ourselves. The parameters will be different if the initial conditions change. For example, if we wish to play a forehand drive in tennis and we are stationary the response parameters will be different from those if we are running across court. Or if we want to kick a soccer ball hard at the goal, the parameters will be different from those if we want to pass it softly to a team-mate. We do not need to have experienced the exact initial conditions or response parameters previously. If a recall schema has been developed, the CNS can automatically adjust the interaction between the two.

Similarly, with the recognition schema, we remember the desired outcome, initial conditions and the sensory consequences. It is the latter that are the most important for the recognition schema. The sensory consequences are what the movement feels like. As with the recall schema, we do not need to have experienced the exact same sensory consequences to know if we are doing the movement as desired. The development of the schema allows us to know if we are within the correct boundaries. Those of you who play striking games, like tennis, cricket, golf or baseball, will all have known that a strike was good, without having to see where the ball went, just from the feel of the movement. You also know when you have underhit or overhit a shot.

The development of the schemas is controlled by *error labelling*. For fast movements sensory information is fedback to the CNS, after the completion of the action. Any mismatches between the desired and actual outcomes are labelled as being errors and are used to alter the schemas, ready for the next time the individual needs to achieve the desired goal. This, also, occurs for slow movements until the recognition schema has been developed, then the sensory information is fedback to the CNS and the movement is continually altered during performance, in order to achieve the desired outcome.

Developing schemas is dependent on the variety of practice. It is not possible to develop schemas if the initial response parameters and sensory consequences remain unaltered. We need to examine a variety of different conditions. As a result, Schmidt examined the concept of *variability of practice*. This is covered in some detail in the next chapter; suffice it to say here that there is strong evidence to support Schmidt's argument that we need to practice with a variety of different initial conditions in order to develop recall and recognition schemas. Also, Schmidt believes that *it is good to make mistakes when learning*. If we only experience success, our schemas will be underdeveloped, particularly the sensory consequences. In other words, if we have not experienced failure, we will be confused by the sensory consequences when the actual movement is not exactly the same as the desired action. However, if we have experienced failure, we will know that what we are feeling is incorrect and will also know what parameters we need to change in order to make the necessary alterations.

Observational Learning Theory

Bandura's (1977) Observational Learning Theory is not an attempt to replace other learning theories but is more an explanation of how we learn from observing demonstrations. It has its origin in social psychology and is primarily concerned with social interaction. However, it has been adapted to motor learning and is often referred to in the skill acquisition literature. According to Bandura, we learn by the *observation of the behaviour of others and the consequences of that behaviour*. Bandura believes that this observation can be *deliberate or incidental*. Deliberate observation is when we explicitly, or overtly, attend to the action being demonstrated. Whether the demonstration is given by a coach for us to copy or whether it is something we see someone doing. Incidental observation is probably how we learn implicitly. We are not overtly aware of observing the skill but nevertheless we do become able to perform it.

In the section on demonstration, we discussed the choice of demonstrator – the coach or a peer or a star performer. According to Bandura, the higher the status of the demonstrator, or model, the more likely the action is to be copied. Research into teaching motor skills does not always support this, as we have seen.

To Bandura, the key to successful observational learning is *reinforcement*. If the model is reinforced, the observer is most likely to imitate the movement. Therefore, if the person sees that the action brings success, they will try to do it themselves. However, if the model is unsuccessful, they are unlikely to copy it. This is self-evident but Bandura found with social behaviour that unsuccessful behaviour is sometimes learnt even though the learner has consciously rejected it. This has major implications for learners because it means that exposure to incorrect movements, in the early stages of learning, may result in the acquisition of bad habits. This supports the point, made in the section on demonstrations, that the model must be able to perform the skill correctly.

Bandura stresses the advantages of the use of *mental imagery and verbal coding* when acquiring skills. He also points out the need to observe complex skills several times before imitation is possible. From what we have said so far, it may look as though Bandura is saying that all we need to do is observe a skill a number of times and then we will be able to repeat it; in fact, he is not. For a skill to be learnt, Bandura asserted that physical practice is essential. Mental imagery can aid learning but cannot replace what Bandura calls *motoric reproduction*.

Dynamical Systems Theory and learning

To the Information Processing theorists, learning is about developing memory and is primarily a function of the CNS. To the ecological psychologists, memory is of little use in the leaning of motor skills. We have no recourse to memory while performing skills. All we need from the CNS is to know what goal we wish to achieve. We then search the environment for the affordance that allows us to achieve our goal. We do not need a motor program or any other central representation to allow us to perform the necessary movement. This is taken care of by the interaction between the environment and ourselves. Until recently, the ecological psychologists rarely talked about learning, although it is difficult to separate many of the arguments of Vygotsky (1978), concerning the development of skills in childhood, from what most psychologists would call learning. Recently, however, ecological psychologists – particularly those following Dynamical Systems Theory – have written and experimented on learning.

To the Dynamical Systems theorists, the key to learning is to *become attuned to affordances*. As perception and action are coupled, once we are able to perceive the affordances we will act automatically. Once the person has decided what goal they want to achieve, they explore the environment to find the affordance. This will occur naturally by *trial and error*. It could be argued that this is the way most of the skills we use today were originally acquired. This is particularly the case in sports where the actual movement used is not the most natural. For example, if we had never seen someone throw a discus we would probably use a very different technique to the one used today. The Ancient Greeks must have worked out the method that the modern technique is based on. By trial and error they found a technique that achieved the goal better than any other. It was obviously good because it is basically the same as the method that is used today.

Taken to its logical conclusion, all the coach would need to do would be to set the goal for the learner. By experimentation, the learner would eventually become attuned to the affordance. This may, of course, be very time consuming. It can also be dangerous with some skills. Many of the safety methods, used by climbers today, were implemented after early climbers saw their colleagues killed. The major role of the instructor is to help the learner to perceive the affordances. The instructor, however, must be aware that what may be an affordance for them may not be for the learner. To the Dynamical Systems theorists, the best way of instructing someone is not to say 'do this' but to guide the learner toward perceiving the affordances for themselves. This is almost analogous to what learning psychologists call *guided discovery*.

Whether using trial and error or guided discovery, the factors that affect learning are task, environmental and organismic constraints. The way in which a cricket ball is bowled today came about directly from the effect of environmental constraints. Early cricketers bowled underarm. This, however, was fairly slow but continued to be the norm until women's fashion changed in the 18th Century. The introduction of skirts with many petticoats meant that it was difficult for the women to bowl underarm. They, therefore, developed roundarm bowling. This was much faster than underarm and was, therefore, soon taken up by men. From this overarm bowling developed.

Bowling, in cricket, is also a good example of how a task constraint affects learning. The rules of cricket mean that the elbow must be locked for most of the bowling action. This will have a major effect on self-organization of the movement. The other constraints that can affect learning are organismic constraints. Although these cannot be easily manipulated, they do affect the way in which the movement is undertaken. Changes in physique result in a change in the way we move. Such changes happen particularly with children but can also occur with adults. Increases in muscle mass due to weight training or weight loss due to dieting all affect the self-organization of the movement.

Another factor is motivation. A form of motivation, described by Vygotsky, is *'bootstrapping'*. Bootstrapping means stretching the learner beyond what they can already do. In other words, the instructor manipulates the constraints so that the learner must acquire a new skill or a new dimension of an old skill in order to achieve their goal.

One of the effects of bootstrapping is what Turvey calls *'freezing' and 'unfreezing' the degrees of freedom.* When we first learn a skill, it is difficult to control the many muscles and joints which are used. As a result, we naturally overcome this by freezing many of the degrees of freedom, e.g., we ensure that some joints are kept locked. Watch someone learning to serve in table tennis. They will lock their wrists and limit the movement of their elbow. When they become proficient, however, they realize that simply getting the ball across the net is not good enough. They must apply spin. This is not possible if the wrists are locked and the elbow is rigid. At this stage the learner must 'unfreeze' the degrees of freedom in order to perform the task properly. For example, in order to impart backspin, the wrist must be loose so that the bat can be swept underneath the centre of the ball. Golfers provide a good example of freezing and 'unfreezing' degrees of freedom. Beginners try hard to keep muscles and joints still so that they do not slice or hook the ball. Experts will deliberately allow free movement of specific joints so that they can deliberately make the ball alter its trajectory in mid-air.

Developmental factors affecting learning

In this section, we briefly examine some of the developmental factors which affect learning. It is not in the scope of this text to examine these areas in detail.

Readers who wish to pursue these topics further should do so in social psychology and developmental textbooks.

Cognitive development

A major factor affecting learning is the learner's stage of cognitive development. The most widely cited cognitive developmental theorist is undoubtedly Jean Piaget. Piaget (1952, 1969) claimed that cognitive development occurred through a process he termed 'adaptation'. Adaptation is an intellectualization of the individual's need to make adjustments with respect to their interaction with the environment. It comes about through the processes of 'accommodation' and 'assimilation'. Accommodation is when the person adjusts responses to meet the specific demands of a new situation, while assimilation is the incorporation of new information into previously-learned cognitive structures. Changes are believed to occur in determined stages.

Piaget identified four stages of development: the sensorimotor phase (birth to 2 years), preoperational thought phase (2 to 7 years), concrete operations phase (7 to 11 years) and the formal operations phase (11 years onward). As we are concerned primarily with skill acquisition from school age to old age, we will concentrate on the last three stages. In the preoperational thought phase the child is interested in 'why' and 'how' things occur. The understanding of this is not through mental processes but through physically manipulating objects. In the next stage of cognitive development, the concrete operations stage, the child moves forward but his/her mental operations are still based on physical manipulations. The key issues are the use of rules for thinking, the ability to differentiate between appearance and reality, and the principle of reversibility, i.e., the capacity of the child to understand that changes in the display can be reversed to their original positions. This capacity allows the child to think through a series of events or actions, and as such he/she can understand what happened and why. According to Piaget, perception, at this stage, is much more developed than at the preoperational thought stage.

Cognition at this stage, however, is still fairly simple. It consists of being able to respond to what the present display affords. There is no attempt to manipulate the display to achieve personal goals. This does not occur until the formal operations stage. In this stage, the person develops a systematic approach to problem solving. Perhaps more importantly, deduction by hypothesis solving and judgement by implication allow the individual to restructure the environment in his/her mind. This enables the performer to be innovative.

These cognitive developmental factors have a major bearing on the learning of decision making. Children in Piaget's preoperational thought stage can master fairly simple decisions. Simple one versus one type tasks provide the child with a display that is not too demanding and the type of decisions require the child to think in simple terms, e.g., in tennis, if there is a space to my opponent's left, I can hit the ball into that space. If we follow the principle of bootstrapping, the child must be introduced to new problems once the simple ones are mastered. If we move to two versus two games, the child has to deal with more perceptual information. This, in itself, should lead to advances in the domain of perception, as the environment forces the child to interact in a more sophisticated manner than in the one versus one situation. However, without intervention from the coach or teacher, advances in decision making may not occur. Without help the child may not be able to determine what is relevant and what is irrelevant information. With help, however, such tasks are within the capability of children in the preoperational stage.

Children in the preoperational stage can see that, when playing in a singles game of tennis, if you hit the ball straight to your opponent they are more likely to return it than if you hit it to one side or the other. Children in the concrete operations stage can go further. They understand that, if you hit the ball to one side, your opponent will have to move to that side in order to return the ball. Furthermore, they can see that, if the opponent is unable to get back into the centre of the court when the ball is returned, they can hit it into the space vacated by their opponent and win the point. Even in more complex team games, e.g., basketball and hockey, they are able to understand that it is better to pass the ball to an unmarked team-mate than to one who is marked. They can also understand defensive duties such as marking an opponent when the opposition has the ball. However, at this stage the child is still making decisions in a simplistic way, responding to the present display rather than thinking ahead and working on strategies to defeat the opposition. At the formal operations stage, the child should be introduced to more complex displays and decisions should require more in the way of cognitive restructuring skills, e.g., the use of decoy runs, in Rugby or basketball, to create space for others.

Although there is little empirical evidence to support Piagetian theory, which is based on observational and interview data, Information Processing Theories of cognitive development are based on empirical data. Much research has been carried out which compares different age groups in the performance of tasks that measure the different factors that make up the Information Processing model, e.g., perception, STM and reaction time. Like Piaget, Information Processing theorists give approximate chronological ages which correspond to when changes in information-processing capacity occur. Similar to Piaget, some accept that, if a child has considerable experience in a specific activity, a particular area could be better developed than others. Research into developmental aspects of perception has shown that static and dynamic visual acuity, depth perception and figure–ground perception (the ability to visually disembed an object from its background) all demonstrate periods of improvement from early childhood until the age of 12 years.

The proficiency of STM in children has been examined by a number of researchers. As we saw in Chapter 6, even in adults STM has severe capacity limitations. While adults can handle 7 ± 2 bits of information, children's limitations are much more severe. Juan Pascual-Leone (1989) claims that by 3 years old the child can handle one bit of information. Every 2 years, from then on, the child adds one more bit; 15-year olds would be at the adult stage. Adults overcome the capacity problems by utilizing strategies such as chunking (see Chapter 6). Chunking can be used by children as young as 5 years old, but only if the child is shown how to do so. Spontaneous chunking is thought to develop at about 9 years old. Spontaneous adult type rehearsal also occurs at about the age of 9 years. This has particular importance in the child's ability to develop a significant LTM store, because without rehearsal the information will not transfer from STM to LTM. It is this limited LTM store that causes the most problems for the child in processing information. It has particularly inhibiting effects on decision making. If decision making depends on the person's ability to compare the present situation with past experiences stored in LTM, then a poor LTM store must hamper decision making. Furthermore, the limited LTM store severely affects selective attention and anticipation. Due to limited past experience, the child is not able to differentiate between relevant and irrelevant stimuli and therefore processes a lot of information which is irrelevant. Similarly, the child is unable to recognize patterns of movement which would allow him/her to anticipate the actions of others, as the child has no memory of similar actions observed in the past.

Cognitive and ecological psychology theories of cognitive development are remarkably similar. They accept that a person may be at a higher or lower stage in any given domain or area of activity, at any specific time, but overall the individual will be at a recognizable stage of development. Moreover, they accept that the genetic potential of the person, at any given age, will impose limitations on how far the individual can progress.

Both schools place great emphasis on the interaction between the individual and the environment. An environment rich in opportunities, for skilled performance, is likely to lead the child to attempt to acquire skills. Mozart is a good example of this. His home was full of opportunities to play musical instruments and his father insisted that he practise from a very early age. The

Williams sisters, in tennis, and Tiger Woods, in golf, are good examples from the world of sport.

So far, we have concentrated on development throughout childhood and adolescence. We need, also, to examine the effect of ageing on cognitive functioning. Generally cognition shows an improvement from adolescence to early adulthood (early to mid-20s). There is then a gradual decline through the middle adulthood years, followed by a rapid decline during old age. The timing of the beginning of this rapid decline varies dramatically between people, therefore it is not possible to delineate chronologically. The decline is caused by structural changes in the brain, due to a loss of CNS neurons. An active lifestyle, mentally and physically, can slow down this loss. A good example of this is Nelson Mandela, who obviously keeps his brain active but, also, exercised every day, even in his 80s. Nevertheless, factors such as reaction time, perception and STM slowly deteriorate. There is, however, some compensation for these losses is the fact that the LTM store increases. Perception is also affected by physical changes such as deterioration in the functioning of the eyes, ears and proprioceptors. Obviously these factors will affect learning capacity. How this happens is discussed in the next section of this chapter.

Motor development

If a person is learning a motor skill, then obviously their stage of motor development will affect that learning. Motor development depends primarily on physical growth and neurophysiological development. Cardiorespiratory factors will also have an effect. Development in these areas begins before birth and continues steadily throughout childhood until puberty. At puberty, there is a sudden increase in development. This lasts for about 4 years. There are great variations in when puberty begins and the length of time it lasts. Girls normally reach puberty at about 11 years old and boys 1–2 years later. Before puberty, there are few gender differences, although girls are generally more flexible than boys. This remains so throughout life. Following puberty, development steadies and continues until about 18 years. There is then a stable period before the ageing process begins (this pre-supposes that the individual does not have an active lifestyle). This is, at first, gradual but there can be dramatic increases in later years. The differences in timing between individuals' ageing processes can be great.

Puberty sees gender changes which have a major effect on the way in which males and females perform some skills. Boys' strength increases dramatically during puberty, whereas girls' improves less. Girls also increase in adipose tissue, which results in differences in cardiorespiratory performance. Both boys and girls increase muscle mass, but boys do so more than girls. Nevertheless, these changes, in both genders, mean that there are alterations in factors, such as centre of gravity, which will affect motor learning.

David Gallahue and John Ozmun put forward a model of stages of motor development (see Figure 8.6). The two early stages are not of interest to us as they occur before children begin learning sports skills. In the *fundamental movement phase*, from 2 to 7 years, children learn to perform 'a variety of

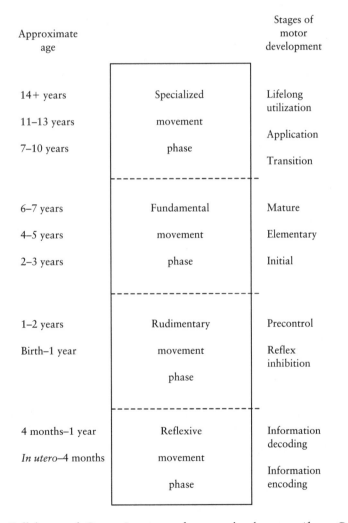

Figure 8.6 Gallahue and Ozmun's stages of motor development (from Gallahue and Ozmun, 1995)

stabilizing, locomotor and manipulative movements, first in isolation then in combination with one another. ... They are gaining increased control in the performance of discrete, serial and continuous movements...' (Gallahue and Ozmun, 1995). The ability to combine facets of a movement is an important one and can be seen in the way children develop the quality of their motor output as they develop in this stage.

During the *specialized movement phase*, the individual develops the basic movements of previous phases into specific actions. Up to the age of about 14 years, the child is learning to apply fundamental movements patterns to complex skills. Whether or not this process will continue to be developed in adulthood will depend on the motivation of the person. Gallahue and Ozmun believe that adults will attempt to develop those skills at which they perceive themselves to be good, but not those at which they think they are poor.

Motor performance begins to deteriorate at some stage in adulthood. When, exactly, will differ greatly from person to person. Research provides us with some very general rules. Strength appears to be at its peak between 25 and 30 years. There is then a very slow decline until about 50 years, followed by a rapid decline. The visual, proprioceptive and cardiorespiratory systems follow similar patterns. However, deterioration can be slowed if the person takes part in physical activity. How well older people can do is remarkable. The World Record for 100 m for 70-year old men is 13.0 s, for 50-year olds it is a remarkable 11.2 s, while the record for 40-year olds, 10.6 s, is better than many club runners are capable of achieving.

Optimal periods of learning

Both Piagetian and ecological psychologists believe that it is not possible to separate cognitive and socioemotional aspects of development. Moreover, these will in turn be affected by physical and motor development. It has long been thought that there are periods at which the interaction between development in each of these areas is ideal for the person to learn. These times are known as *critical periods of learning*. The term 'critical' is based on animal studies. When animals do not learn a particular skill at the critical time, they either do not acquire it at all or acquire a very inferior version. Something similar happens with humans but not as severely and we can learn at a time after the critical period. As a result Robert Singer (1968) coined the phrase '*optimal periods of learning*'. This is a more accurate description.

Practical implications

It is easy for psychologists, engaged in the study of learning, to become engrossed in the theoretical aspects of the phenomenon and forget that the idea of studying learning is to provide the learner and teacher with guidelines for bringing about successful skill acquisition. In this section, we examine some practical applications of issues which we have covered in this chapter. We will take these further in the following chapter, after we have examined the nature of practice.

The first issue facing the coach or teacher is what to teach to any particular group of individuals. In order to decide, the coach must take into account a number a key factors. First of all, he/she should try to ascertain the type and level of motivation possessed by the group. This is not all that simple. Few coaches have access to psychometric tests of motivation; moreover, such tests are open to the learner telling the coach what they think he/she wants to hear. In reality, the coach must decide what the athlete's type and level of motivation is, based on observation. This may involve a great deal of trial and error. Just observing how the learners respond to different types of instruction will provide a lot of clues. This aspect of coaching is sometimes described as being an art. I would rather think of it as being a skill. By calling it an art we imply that it cannot be learnt but, in fact, it can. The more experienced you become, the better you are able to detect motivational types and levels.

Another way to determine motivation is to include the learners in the setting of goals. These can be *group goals* or *individual goals* or both. If coaches include the learner or learners in this process, they will get some idea of what the learners want. Moreover, the goals will belong to the learners as much as they do to the coach. If coaches set the goals themselves, they are the coaches' goals not the athletes'. Goals should be *challenging*, i.e., they should lead to bootstrapping. They should, in other words, inspire the learner to stretch beyond current boundaries. Although they should be challenging, they must also be *attainable*. If the learner thinks 'I will never be able to do that', they are very unlikely to even try.

Goals need to be both *long-term* and *short-term*. Long-term goals are what they say they are, what you are aiming for in the long term. This time span may be anything from a few weeks to a year or more. With most of my teams, we set goals for the end of the season or even for the beginning of the following season. Short-term goals should be stepping-stones to the long-term goals. It is important with short-term goals that the learner can obtain success. Also, learners need to have some way of *measuring* whether or not they are achieving their goals. This does not have to be objective or quantitative measuring; it can be a subjective assessment of performance. However, it does help if some quantitative value is given. With my soccer teams when we have set goals about improving positional play, for example, I gave each player a mark out of ten at the end of each game. Thus, they could see how they were doing. One of the problems with short-term goals is that one does not always achieve them and sometimes extraneous circumstances intervene. As a result, we need to be able to change our goals, particularly our short-term goals. They need to be *flexible*.

Most of the literature about goals suggests that we should set *performance* goals. These are goals concerning the quality of the performance. However, recent research suggests that we should also set *outcome* goals. These are goals regarding our performance with respect to others, e.g., we will win the league or a particular championship. I had a good example of the use of goal setting with an 11-year old school soccer team. Our long-term goals, for the season, were keeping possession of the ball for more than three passes and to pressure the opposition so that we let in no more than one goal a game. In that season, we won only one game. However, the boys' individual and group performances steadily improved and at the end of the season both they and I were happy. In the next two seasons, we won the league and the cup and lost only two games.

As well as taking into account motivation, the coach needs to be aware of the cognitive and developmental stages of his/her group or individual. Chronological age is helpful but, as we have seen, different individuals develop at different rates. More importantly the stage of development of an individual in a particular activity might be very different from their overall developmental stage. While this tends to occur more with children, it can also occur with older age groups. For example, the ski instructor cannot simply look at a class and decide 'well they are all about 40, so I had better not expect too much from them physically'. Many 40-year olds are fitter than many 20-year olds. With children, however, knowledge of such factors as STM limitations, reaction time and selective attention can be very useful.

With such information in mind, the coach can decide what skills the group or individual should learn. Also, coaches can determine the way in which they are going to instruct. How much verbal and visual information can they give? This is particularly important because many coaches overload the individual's STM. With regard to older age groups, it appears that the older the person, the more information they want before trying the skill for themselves. While children are willing to 'have a go', even without any instruction, older people want all the information they can get before trying out the skill. It would appear that they want declarative knowledge before they try to obtain procedural knowledge. I saw a graphic example of this several years ago. I observed Ken Illingworth, a lawn bowls coach and former England international, coach a group of 10-year olds then a group of over 60s. With the children, he let them have a go without any instruction. Chaos ruled. There were woods (the technical name for the bowl) going everywhere. Everyone had a laugh and then Ken was able to show the children how to bowl properly. He kept instructions to a minimum and kept the children active. With the adults, he explained everything in detail but still some wanted even more instruction before trying for themselves. A different approach, but by the end of the two sessions both groups had learnt about the same amount.

We will return to the practical implications of theory and research into learning at the end of the next chapter. Suffice it to say, for now, that knowledge of cognitive and motor development and how individuals learn should guide the coach's choice of what to coach and how to coach it.

Key points

- Learning is a relatively permanent change in performance resulting from practice or experience.

- Learning can be explicit or implicit:

  - explicit learning is when we consciously set out to acquire skill and/or knowledge,

  - implicit learning takes place subconsciously without intent.

- We cannot directly measure learning, we can only infer its presence by measuring performance.

- 'Learning' can be measured by:

  - retention tests – a test of performance following a period of no practice,

  - transfer tests – performance of the skill in a different environment or situation,

  - measuring performance curves – plotting performance over a period of time.

Information Processing Theory and learning

- Learning is a function of the CNS.

- We can acquire declarative and/or procedural knowledge:

  o declarative knowledge is knowing what to do,

  o procedural knowledge is knowing what to do and how to do it.

- The acquisition of motor skills requires physical rehearsal but:

  o mental rehearsal can aid physical rehearsal,

  o imagery is a particularly powerful form of mental rehearsal.

- Instruction can be verbal, visual or verbal plus visual:

  o verbal plus visual is the most effective,

  o some skills are very difficult to put into words.

- Demonstrations are a particularly useful form of instruction:

  o demonstrations can be given by the coach or by a peer,

  o demonstrations can be motivational as well as instructive.

Cognitivist theories of learning

- Fitts and Posner's Three Stage Theory:

  o cognitive stage – use of verbal labels,

  o associative stage – practice is required to refine the skill,

  o autonomous stage – the skill becomes automatic.

- Gentile's Model:

  o initial acquisition stage – verbalization takes place; learners get the basic idea; selective attention is developed; an action plan is formulated,

  o skill refinement stage – practice leads to fixation and diversification,

  o fixation is the refinement of closed skills,

- diversification is the ability to use movements in an open skill situation.

- Adam's Closed-loop Theory of Learning:

  - we develop a perceptual trace (memory of the feel of past performances),

  - the trace is compared to the movement being undertaken and alterations are made if necessary,

  - we develop a memory trace,

  - the memory trace is responsible for the selection and initiation of movement,

  - development of the traces takes place in the verbal–motor stage and motor stage,

  - in the verbal–motor stage the movement is verbalized but physical practice is also necessary,

  - in the motor stage the movement is automatic and does not require verbalization.

- Schmidt's Schema Theory:

  - recall memory is responsible for the choice and initiation of action,

  - recognition memory evaluates the ongoing movement and makes any necessary changes,

  - recall schemas are based on: the memory of the desired outcome; initial conditions; response parameters (changes in the specifics of the movement if action is to be successful); sensory consequences (what the movement feels like),

  - recognition schemas are based on: the memory of the desired outcome; the initial conditions; sensory consequences.

- Error labelling (comparison of desired and actual outcomes) aids schema formation:

- variability of practice (practising with different initial conditions, thus requiring different response parameters) aids error labelling.

- Observational Learning Theory:

  - observation of others aids learning,

  - observation can be deliberate or incidental,

  - successful actions are copied,

  - mental imagery and verbal coding aid learning,

  - physical practice is essential for the learning of motor skills.

Dynamical systems theory and learning

- Practice in realistic situations helps us to become attuned to affordances (know what parts of the environment to search for opportunities to achieve our goal).

- Learning can take place by trial and error.

- Coaches can help us to perceive the affordances and make the movement efficiently by placing constraints on us:

  - task and environmental constraints 'force' us to learn the most efficient way of performing a skill and/or to perform within the rules of a sport,

  - constraints 'force' us to freeze the degrees of freedom when in the early stages of learning,

  - releasing the constraints or altering them can lead to the refinement of a skill in the later stages of learning.

Cognitive development and learning

- Limitations to cognitive development affect the ability of the individual to learn skills which require much in the way of perception and decision making:

  ○ limitations in selective attention; short-term memory capacity; ability to chunk; ability to use rehearsal; long-term memory store; reaction time; figure–ground perception.

- According to Piaget each stage of development results in limitations in ability to learn:

  ○ in the preoperational stage (2 to 7 years), the child is interested in physically exploring the environment,

  ○ in the concrete operations phase (7 to 11 years), the child can react to changes in the environment but cannot consciously act upon the environment to create changes,

  ○ in the formal operations stage (11+ years), the person can act upon the environment to create opportunities for action and has a systematic approach to problem solving.

Motor development and learning

- The person's physical and neurophysiological state will affect the type of skills they can learn.

- Gallahue and Ozmun identified stages of motor development:

  ○ in the fundamental movement phase (2 to 7 years), the child can learn basic motor movements (e.g., gymnastic skills, swimming strokes),

  ○ in the specialized movement phase (7 to 11 years), these basic skills can be developed into complex skills (e.g., striking a ball with a bat can be developed into cricket, baseball or hockey skills),

  ○ after 14 years, these skills can be refined and reach very high levels if the person continues to practise.

- The point at which ageing begins to affect skill acquisition and performance varies greatly from person to person.

Practical implications

- Coaches should set goals for learners:
  - these should be challenging but obtainable,
  - they can be short- or long-term,
  - performance goals are thought to be better than outcome goals for most people,
  - goals should be measurable,
  - they should be flexible,
  - the learner should be involved in setting the goals.
- Children like to try a skill before receiving detailed instruction.
- Adults like to have detailed instruction before trying a skill.

Test your knowledge

(Answers in Appendix 3.)

Part one

Fill in the blank spaces using words taken from the list below (NB there are more words in the list than there are spaces).

Kerr (1982) defined learning as being a relatively _____ change in performance, resulting from _____ or _____. Performance, on the other hand, _____ from time to time. We cannot directly measure learning, we can only _____ it based on _____. Learning is measured by retention tests. The amount that has been learned is said to be demonstrated by the amount that is retained over a period of _____. Another method of measuring learning is transfer tests. The use of transfer tests is based on the assumption that if a task is well learned it can be performed in _____ _____. The third method commonly used to measure learning is the use of performance _____.

When learning some tasks the learner reaches periods when no improvement is shown; these are termed _____. These periods may be caused by _____ _____. Learning can be positive or _____, but is always demonstrated by _____.

plateaus   permanent   negative   no practice   reactive   scores
different   fluctuates inhibition   practice   performance
consistency   graph   experience   curves   environments
infer

Part two

Choose which of the phrases, (a), (b), (c) or (d), best completes the statement or answers the question. There is only *one* correct answer for each problem.

1. Which of the following types of instruction has been shown to be the most effective?

    (a) verbal,

    (b) visual,

    (c) visual plus verbal,

    (d) demonstration.

2. If a coach wants his/her athletes to learn from a demonstration, he/she should be careful:

    (a) not to show off when demonstrating,

    (b) to do the demonstration slowly so that the athletes can see what is happening,

    (c) to point out the key points to be looked at,

    (d) to show how to do the skill wrongly as well as correctly.

3. Adams's (1971) perceptual trace is the same as:

    (a) Schmidt's (1975) recall memory,

    (b) Schmidt's (1975) recognition memory,

    (c) Gentile's (1972) fixation,

(d) Gentile's (1972) diversification.

4. According to Schmidt (1975), when learning it is useful to:

    (a) avoid errors,

    (b) make errors,

    (c) carry out very specific practice,

    (d) use blocked practice.

5. According to Bandura (1977), we are most likely to copy the performance of:

    (a) a friend,

    (b) a coach,

    (c) someone our own age,

    (d) a star performer.

6. According to Bandura (1977), which of the following is *essential* for learning to take place?

    (a) mental imagery,

    (b) mental rehearsal,

    (c) verbal coding,

    (d) physical practice.

7. According to Vygotsky (1978), bootstrapping is:

    (a) stretching the learner beyond their current boundaries,

    (b) freezing the degrees of freedom,

    (c) unfreezing the degrees of freedom,

    (d) controlling self-organization.

8. Children will be unlikely to be able to perceive the need for, and use of, decoy runs in team games until they:

    (a) are in Piaget's concrete operations stage,

(b) are in Piaget's formal operations stage,

(c) reach adulthood,

(d) can handle 5 ± 2 bits of information.

Part three

Below are a number of questions (Q) and answers (A). Fill in the spaces using the phrases below.

1. Q. What do we call a performance curve that demonstrates a great deal of learning in the early stages then _____?

   A. A negatively accelerated curve.

2. Q. What do we call a _____?

   A. A plateau.

3. Q. What did Anderson (1982) call _____?

   A. Declarative knowledge.

4. Q. What did Anderson (1982) call _____?

   A. Procedural knowledge

5. Q. What do we call _____?

   A. Implicit learning.

6. Q. What is the most common form of _____?

   A. Mental imagery.

7. Q. Which group of psychologists believed that humans learn _____?

   A. The Gestältists.

8. Q. In which phase of learning do Fitts and Posner (1967) claim that we _____?

A. Cognitive phase.

9. Q. According to Gentile (1972), what is developed when the learner is able _____?

A. Selective attention

10. Q. Which of Gentile's (1972) stages of learning is characterized by _____?

A. Skill-refinement stage.

11. Q. Which of Adams' (1971) learning stages is similar to Fitts and Posner's _____?

A. The motor stage.

12. Q. According to Schmidt (1975), what kind of memory _____?

A. Recognition memory.

13. Q. In developing the recall schema, we remember the _____. What name did Schmidt (1975) give to this?

A. Response parameters.

14. Q. Which part of the recognition schema allows us to remember _____?

A. Sensory consequences.

15. Q. Why did Schmidt (1975) say that it is best to _____?

A. It allows us to experience different initial response parameters and sensory consequences.

16. Q. What does Turvey (1992) say that we should do when learning a new skill in order to control _____?

A. Freeze the degrees of freedom.

mental rehearsal
changes in the specifics of the action
use variable practice
knowing what to do
by problem solving
the movement of muscles and joints
autonomous stage
to differentiate between relevant and irrelevant cues
learning sub-consciously

evaluates the ongoing movement
what the movement feels like
use verbal labelling
slows down
period of no apparent learning
fixation and diversification
knowing what to do and how to do it

Part four

Which of the following statements are true (T) and which are false (F)?

1. Piaget's preoperational stage of development lasts from
    2–7 years.   T   F

2. Children in Piaget's preoperational phase can successfully
    play two versus two games.   T   F

3. Children in Piaget's concrete operations stage can use decoy
    runs in team games.   T   F

4. According to Pascual-Leone (1989), a child increases his/her
    mental capacity by 1 bit of information every 3 years.   T   F

5. Children have relatively poor selective attention because of
    limitations in short-term memory.   T   F

6. A child cannot be outstanding at one sport but only average
    at other sports.   T   F

7. Girls' strength increases at puberty.   T   F

8. Girls are more flexible than boys.   T   F

9. Gallahue and Ozmun's (1995) fundamental movement phase
    covers the same ages as Piaget's preoperational phase.   T   F

10. According to Gallahue and Ozmun (1995), children will
    continue to develop motor skills after the age of 14 years only
    if they are motivated.   T   F

11. Undertaking physical activity will not slow the ageing process. T   F

12.	Optimal periods of learning occur when the person is mentally, physically and emotionally ready to learn.	T	F
13.	Goals should lead to bootstrapping.	T	F
14.	Once a goal has been set, we should never change it.	T	F
15.	Performance goals are about how we compare with others.	T	F
16.	Older adults need less instruction than children.	T	F

Additional reading

Gallahue DL and Ozmun JC (1995) *Understanding motor development*, Brown & Benchmark, Madison, Wisconsin, USA

Turpin BAM (1982) Enhancing skill acquisition through application of information processing. *Motor Skills: Theory into Practice* **6**: 77–83

Williams LRT (2001) On movement coordination: some implications for teaching and learning. *J Intl Council for Health, Physical Education, Recreation, Sport, and Dance* **37**: 17–22

9 Practice

Learning Objectives

By the end of this chapter, you should be able to

♦ understand and classify different types of practice

♦ understand the nature and effect of contextual interference

♦ understand the nature and effect of variability of practice

♦ understand how and why transfer of training works

♦ define and classify feedback

♦ understand the role of feedback in the retention of skills

♦ understand how Dynamical Systems Theory accounts for the effect of practice with particular reference to

◊ the use of constraints

◊ attunement to affordances

♦ understand the implications for coaches and performers

Acquisition and Performance of Sports Skills   T. McMorris
© 2004 John Wiley & Sons, Ltd   ISBNs: 0-470-84994-0 (HB); 0-470-84995-9 (PB)

Introduction

Practice is a major, if not *the* major, part of learning. I have separated learning and practice, in this book, simply in order to make it easier to follow. In reality, we cannot separate the one from the other. To the cognitivists, practice follows instruction. It is the key factor in Fitts and Posner's intermediate and autonomous stages, Adams' motor stage and Gentile's skill refinement stage. Anderson would see it as being when we move from declarative knowledge (knowing what to do) to procedural knowledge (developing the ability to perform the task). To the Dynamical Systems theorists *practice is learning*.

Information Processing Theory and practice

Types of practice

In this section, we will examine the main types of practice which have been highlighted by researchers and theorists. In doing this, however, we must be aware that the vast majority of research into practice has been with tasks that are not ecologically valid. Nevertheless, much of the information is useful. Where ecological validity is an issue, we will examine it.

Massed and spaced practice

One of the first areas of practice to be examined was massed versus spaced practice. Technically, massed practice is defined as practice where the intervals between trials of the task are less than the time it takes to complete one trial. In reality, massed practice is practice where there is little or no gap between trials. Spaced practice, in its literal sense, is where the interval between the trials is greater than the time it takes for one trial to be completed. In reality, it is when practice is interspersed with rest periods or breaks. Research has generally shown that there is no difference in learning resulting from the two types of practice. Spaced practice can sometimes lead to better performance because either boredom (reactive inhibition) or fatigue can set in during massed practice. Following a rest, however, there is no difference when retention tests are conducted.

While many textbooks suggest that spaced practice should be used when the task is fatiguing, some coaches like to practice when fatigue has set in. Fatigue often results in performers changing the dynamics of the movement, yet they still achieve the goals. In sports where skills have to be performed while in a fatigued state, this type of practice can be desirable. Coaches should not be afraid of having their athletes practise while fatigued because research has shown that *fatigue does not affect learning*. After a rest, the person is able to perform the task as well as the individual who learned it in a non-fatigued condition. Environmental factors such as heat, cold and rain etc. have a similar effect. They affect performance but not learning.

While the evidence is that neither massed nor spaced practice is the better with regard to learning, the coach should be aware of motivational effects. To many learners, massed practice is less enjoyable, as they become bored with repeating the same task over and over again without a break. On the other hand, some performers feel that breaks are a waste of time and that they could be doing something useful in the time between practices. It is up to the coach and players to agree what is best for them.

Whole and part practice

Very little ecologically valid research has been carried out into the use of whole and part practice. Nevertheless, theoretical underpinnings for which is the more likely to produce the better results do exist. It is not, however, a simple case of one type of practice being better than the other. The nature of the task, the experience and developmental stage of the learners all effect which type of practice will lead to optimal results. Moreover, the definitions 'whole' and 'part' are somewhat ambiguous. Whole practice can apply, as the word implies, to practising a task in its entirety; but what is its entirety? Playing a game is certainly whole practice; but what about practising a team game, e.g., hockey, in a *small-sided game*. I have seen this classed as both whole and part practice by different psychologists. The best explanation of whether it is whole or part is probably how it relates to the learner. For an adult, playing six-a-side hockey is not whole practice. For an 11-year old, however, it can be classed as whole practice because the level of development of the 11-year old means that playing 11-a-side is not an appropriate task.

The situation with regard to the definition of part practice is even more complicated. The strictest definition of part practice would be practising a part of a skill in isolation to the rest of the task. For example, a triple jumper might practise the hop phase only. Another explanation of part practice is practising a skill in a non-game situation. Tennis players practise volleying, with the coach serving them. This is normally called part practice, but it is nearer to whole practice than the triple jumper working just on the hop phase.

A particular kind of part practice is *part-progressive practice* and it is this that is the most commonly used of all the types of practice. Part-progressive practice is when the task is broken down into parts and the individual practises part one, then adds part two, followed by part three and so on. Bowling in cricket is normally practised in this way. The learner practises the ball release standing still, not moving their feet. They, then, do the same but transfer their weight from being on the back foot to the front foot. They then take a step forward before bowling. This is followed by adding the run up. Thus, the parts are added together to form a whole. I am sure that you will all have encountered this type of practice. Coaching manuals are full of such examples; but what are the advantages and disadvantages of each of these types of practice?

In order to answer this question, we must refer back to what we have learned about the nature of skill, the way in which we make decisions and the limitations of the person's CNS. Whole practice has the advantage of putting the skill in the environment in which it is to be used. Not only does the learner practise the technique but also learns *how* and *when* to use that particular technique. In other words, whole practice develops not only technique but also decision making. To the cognitivists, whole practice is also good in helping the learner to develop schemas. They cannot simply repeat a specific motor program.

Whole practice, however, can have major drawbacks. This can be particularly so when learning team games. The amount of stimuli that the learner must deal with, when playing a full version of a game, can be overwhelming for the beginner, particularly if the learner is a child, with limited selective attention and past experience. Even where the perceptual and decision-making demands are not too great, whole practice can be difficult if the motor-control demands are exacting. We have looked at bowling in cricket. The nature of this task, particularly the fact that it is an unnatural movement, means that it can be hard for beginners to do without breaking it down.

From what we have seen in the previous paragraphs, you will no doubt have worked out that the advantage of part practice is that it places less stress on the individual's perceptual, decision-making and motor-control faculties. However, two major problems arise. If we subdivide a skill into its parts, we need eventually to put the parts together to form the whole. This often causes problems and leads to the performance curve plateauing or even reversing. Part-progressive practice is a way of overcoming this. As we saw with the cricket bowling, we can gradually build up the skill. The other problem is that practising in isolation means that the learner does not have to decide when or where to use the skill in the real situation. The tennis player learning to volley does not only need to know the techniques of volleying but when to volley and which volleying technique to use in any given situation. This can be overcome to some extent in part-progressive practice. The progressions can include the introduction of opposition. The cricket bowler can begin bowling at the stumps without a batter. The batter can be added as a progression. The tennis player can be given targets to aim at, which can only be hit if different techniques are used. The Rugby coach will often begin practising a skill unopposed, add static opposition and in the later stages increase the activity of the opposition. Even adding co-operating players can be a progression. In Figure 9.1(a), we can see that the goalkeeper does not have to make a decision about whether to go and catch the cross or not, he is the only defender therefore he must go. In Figure 9.1(b), however, a decision needs to be made. Does he go for the cross or leave it to his defender?

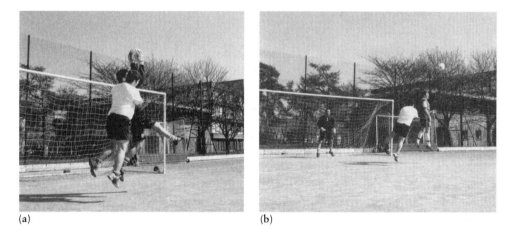

(a)   (b)

Figure 9.1 Example of part-progressive practice in order to coach decision making: in the first practice (a), the goalkeeper is the only defender, therefore his decision of whether to go for the cross or stay on his goal line is limited; in (b) a defender is added and this makes the goalkeeper's decision more complex

Another problem, with using part practice and part-progressive practice, is if the learner does not know where the parts are leading to. This can cause the learner to acquire inappropriate actions. If there is no batter facing the learner bowler, they may bowl very slowly and have the ball bounce in a wrong place. If they are hitting the wicket, however, they think they are doing well. They need to know that such balls are easy for the batter to strike. Not knowing where the practice is leading can also affect motivation. I came across this when teaching Rugby to a class of 13-year old boys. Everything was going fine until I introduced scrummaging. I used the progressions recommended in the coaching manuals, scratch scrums followed by three-man scrums and so on. The boys, who had been very keen, suddenly became somewhat lethargic. One of then plucked up the courage to ask, 'why are we doing this, what has it to do with anything'? I realized then that they did not know where the scrum fitted into the game. I had assumed that 13-year old boys had seen Rugby games played and knew what I was moving towards. When I asked the class of 36 boys who had not seen a proper Rugby game, 33 hands went up.

In order to overcome this problem, *whole–part–whole* practice is recommended in the textbooks. In this, we try the whole briefly in order to see where the task fits in with the real game. Then the practices are broken down into manageable parts. Gradually, we build up to return to the whole. This is not always possible due to the nature of the task. I could not let my boys have a go at scrummaging; it is too dangerous if they have not been instructed in the correct technique. I overcame the problem by showing them a video of the scrum working in a real game.

Pure part practices are rarely used with beginners but are common with experienced performers. If the coach sees that an athlete has a problem with an aspect of performance they will practise that particular part in isolation. The problem of not knowing where it fits into the whole skill is non-existent because of the athlete's level of experience. Also, motivation is not a problem because performers, at this level of sport, know that by getting the part right their overall performance will improve. Even stars like Tiger Woods will use part practice in this way. Linford Christie spent hours developing his sprint start as he saw that as a weakness. This led to him winning an Olympic gold medal. Practice should not only be to correct weaknesses, however; it should also be used to perfect already good skills. Gianfranco Zola, the Italian footballer, practises taking free kicks every day, despite the fact that he is one of the best in the world. Likewise, the England Rugby star Jonny Wilkinson takes 50 place kicks every day, in order to stay the best in the world. Similarly, the world-renowned basketball player 'Magic' Johnson used to take 80 shots at basket before and after training every day.

Based on theory, we can say that, where possible, whole practice should be used. However, if the perceptual and decision-making demands are too great for the learners, we need to use part-progressive practice. Similarly, if the motor-control demands are too much for the learners, we must break the task down into parts. Pure part practice is best used by experienced performers. Notice that, in all cases, we must look at the interaction between the task and the learner. This part of this text is, in fact, a pulling together of the many parts which we have examined in the previous chapters. In order to organize practices properly we must take into account the nature of the skill (Chapter 1), perceptual demands (Chapter 2), decision-making demands (Chapter 3), memory limitations (Chapter 4) and motor-control factors (Chapter 7). We, also, should take into account reaction time (Chapter 5) and anticipation (Chapter 6) because limitations in the development of these will affect the amount of information and the level of motor control that the learner brings to the practice (see Figure 9.2).

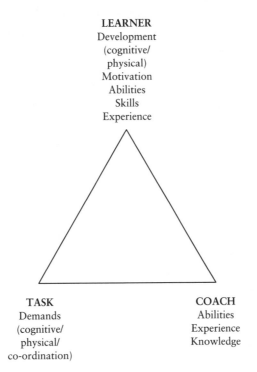

LEARNER
Development
(cognitive/
physical)
Motivation
Abilities
Skills
Experience

TASK
Demands
(cognitive/
physical/
co-ordination)

COACH
Abilities
Experience
Knowledge

Figure 9.2   Factors affecting choice of type of practice

Variability of practice

Variability of practice means practising the skill using a variety of task and environmental demands. We might practise running up and down hill. We may play basketball on courts of different sizes. Mostly variability of practice refers to asking the learner to produce different versions of a task, for example kick the ball 20 m, kick it 30 m, kick it hard, kick it softly and so on. The tennis player may be asked to play shots across court and down the line, while the badminton player may be asked to serve short or long.

To the Information Processing theorists, variability of practice is vital because otherwise we cannot develop schemas and hence build up generalized motor programs. According to Schmidt's Schema Theory, when we use variable practice we alter the initial conditions, response parameters and the sensory consequences. We talked earlier about Gianfranco Zola and Jonny Wilkinson practising kicks. They do not kick from the same place each time. By starting at different angles and distances from the goal, they build up a store of different initial conditions. In order to score, they must alter the response parameters. A long kick requires the application of more power and a longer leg movement. Similarly, the sensory feel of the movement will differ, albeit subtly. It is the ability to recognize these subtle differences that makes such players the stars they are.

Theoretically, there is very strong support for variability of practice. However, research is less supportive. Research with children has generally supported variability. However, with adults it has generally failed to support the theory. It is almost certain that the children are in the developmental process of building up schemas, whereas the adults have probably gone through these processes during their childhood. Therefore, varying practice has less of an effect.

Blocked, random and serial practice

The decision to use blocked, random or serial practice is often referred to as *practice scheduling*. Blocked practice is when the *learner practises one skill continually with no interference from the performance of other skills.* When undertaking random practice the *athlete will perform two or more skills having random trials on each skill.* Serial practice is a version of random practice. The *learner practises more than one skill and practice is interspersed between the skills but in a serial order,* i.e., one skill is practised for a set number of trials, followed by practise on another skill, followed by practise on a third skill and back to the beginning. Then the cycle is repeated.

Common sense says that using blocked practice will be the most beneficial. As we saw in Chapter 6, when looking at the effect of interpolated activity on motor memory, random and serial practice should lead to disruption in learning. This is shown when we examine performance, i.e., when performance is tested immediately following practice, blocked practice results in the best performance. However, when a retention test is undertaken, random and serial practice produce better results than blocked practice. Battig (1979) called this the *contextual interference effect.*

Shea and Morgan (1979) tried to explain these counter-intuitive results by putting forward the theory of *elaboration.* Shea and Morgan argued that, when we practise randomly and serially, we use more strategies to carry out the skill rather than when we stick to one plan as in the blocked situation. Perhaps more importantly, all three skills are held in working memory at the same time, thus allowing the learner to compare recall, recognition and sensory consequences of the skills. Lee and Magill (198) disagreed with this theory and put forward the theory of *action plan reconstruction*. According to them, the learner experiences partial or total forgetting of a skill during the periods when he/she is working on the other skills. On returning to the 'forgotten' skill, they have to re-plan the way in which they will perform it, i.e., re-draw their action plan. This aids the development of schemas. There is no research evidence to support one theory more than the other.

An interesting development on the effect of research into contextual interference has been to show that the effect is not always demonstrated and depends on the type of task. If two or more tasks which are very different are practised then the effect is demonstrated. By 'very different' I mean where they are not using the same generalized motor program. If tasks require variations of the same generalized motor program, the contextual interference effect is not shown. This type of practice is, in fact, no different to variability of practice as discussed in the last section. Variations of the same generalized motor program are tasks like the punch volley, stop volley and drive volley in tennis or the set shot and jump shot in basketball.

Transfer of training

Transfer of training refers to the effect that *practice on one task has on the learning or performance of another task*. I am sure that most of you will have experienced this, to some extent, during your lives. Pat Jennings, the former Northern Ireland, Tottenham and Arsenal goalkeeper, played Gaelic Football at school. Practising catching the ball in Gaelic, with the opposition clamouring all over him, was transferred to professional soccer. There have been some recent examples of Rugby League players transferring to Rugby Union, the most notable being Jason Robinson, while the last British male to win Wimbledon, Fred Perry, also played top-class table tennis. There was no transfer from these activities to making sports shirts, however.

Transfer of this kind is termed *positive transfer* and is defined as being when the practice of one task has *a facilitating effect* on the learning or performance of another. We mostly think of transfer as being positive, similar to the examples I have given above. Transfer can also be *negative*. Negative transfer is defined as being when the practice of one task has an *inhibiting effect* on the learning or performance of another. In my very first game of hockey, I found myself playing a forward defensive cricket shot when trying to stop the ball. It was a good forward defensive shot but of no use to me. The nature of a forward defensive shot meant that my body position was totally inappropriate for playing hockey and my opponent happily ran off with the ball, leaving me stranded and unable to move quickly. Initially, Jason Robinson, while enjoying his move to Rugby Union, sometimes demonstrated negative transfer, doing inappropriate things during a game. The Welsh international, Jonathan Davies suffered similarly when moving to Rugby League from Union.

Whether transfer is negative or positive, it is classed as being either *proactive* or *retroactive*. If transfer is positive, it is known as *proactive or retroactive facilitation*. If it is negative, it is called *proactive or retroactive inhibition*. Proactive transfer is when the practice on a task affects the learning or performance of a *subsequent* task. My forward defensive shot is an example of proactive inhibition, while Jason Robinson's dazzling side-step is an example of proactive facilitation. Retroactive transfer is when practice of one task affects the performance of a *previously learned or practised* task. I commented earlier about my attempts to play table tennis style backhand flicks when playing tennis, particularly at the beginning of the tennis season. This is an example of retroactive inhibition. A good example of retroactive facilitation can be seen when basketball players play netball and then return to basketball. The need in netball to lose your marker often transfers very well to basketball, when the opposition is playing a full court press.

The kind of transfer that we have been talking about, so far, is called *inter-task transfer*, i.e., transfer from one task to another, although our example of Rugby players switching codes is much nearer to *intra-class transfer*. Intra-class transfer is when there is transfer between *variations of the same task*. A hockey player shooting at goal and making a long pass or a tennis player playing a drive volley and a stop volley. A specific form of intra-class transfer is what we call *shaping skills*. Shaping skills is used with learners. The athlete begins with an easy version of the task and moves on to more difficult versions. Figure 9.3 shows an example of this. In Figure 9.3(a), the learners are in twos and have simply to pass the ball to their colleague. In Figure 9.3(b), they are placed into a four versus one game, with the one trying to intercept passes. Thus the task is even more difficult. In Figure 9.3(c), a second defender is added and, in Figure 9.3(d), they have a three versus three game.

This is a case of moving from *simple* to *complex*. Transfer can also occur from *complex* to *simple*. Although simple to complex would appear to offer a greater likelihood of transfer, complex to simple can have startling effects. One of my students, Michelle Coleman, trained two groups of girls on a headspring.

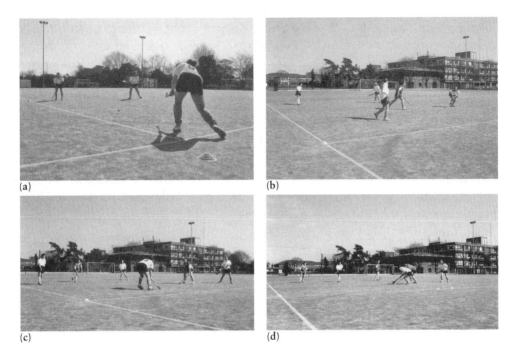

Figure 9.3 Example of developing a skill from easy to hard (a) unopposed passing; (b) four versus one; (c) four versus two; (d) three versus three

The first group practised from simple to hard, they began by using a box to give them more height for landing. The other group started from the ground and later moved to using the box, thus, moving from hard to easy. At the end of 3 weeks of practice, the two groups were tested head springing from the floor and from the box. The group that went from difficult to easy was significantly better than the other group in both conditions. The most likely explanation for this is that, in order to do a head spring from the ground, the girls had to learn to push with their arms and swing their legs through fast, right from the start. Although the simple to complex group gradually progressed to be able to do a headspring without the box, they were not as adept. They had been able to use the box to give them height in the early stages, so were not fully aware of the underlying principles – hence the poorer performance.

One must be careful in deciding when to go from simple to difficult and vice versa. Generally, the principles for deciding are similar to those for determining whether to use whole or part-progressive practice. The coach must know of what his/her athletes are capable. My student was an experienced gymnastics coach and she knew that these girls were capable of going from hard to easy. Moreover, the principles that need to be learned cannot be too demanding.

Where there are a lot of perceptual demands or the neuropsychological demands are exacting for the learners, easy to hard should be used.

Transfer theories

So far, we have talked about negative and positive transfer but have not tried to explain why one would happen rather than the other. Nor have we discussed the fact that sometimes transfer does not occur at all. Before moving on to this, it is probably a good idea to examine some of the theories of transfer. The notion of transfer has been discussed by psychologists for many years. The first to put forward a theory was Judd (1908). Judd's theory is known as the *general elements theory*. Judd believed that positive transfer occurs when two tasks require the same or similar *general principles*. Someone going from playing soccer to hockey will be able to use the same general principles for team play. He also thought that there would be transfer if two tasks used the same *neurological pathways*. For example, throwing a ball will transfer to throwing a javelin. The great Australian cricketer Sir Donald Bradman practised, by himself, for hours throwing a golf ball against a wall and hitting it using a cricket stump. This practice required both the use of general principles and the same neurological pathways.

The second major theory to be put forward to explain transfer was Thorndike's (1927) *identical elements theory*. Looking at the title this would appear to be very different from Judd's general elements theory, in fact it would appear to be the opposite. On closer inspection, however, they do not differ very much. Thorndike's use of the words 'element' and 'identical' is somewhat different from the way most people would use them. According to Thorndike, transfer would occur if the purposes of two responses were the same regardless of the nature of the stimulus. So he would expect positive transfer between an overhead smash in tennis and badminton, even though the stimuli (ball versus shuttlecock) and the actual nature of the shots (wrist comparatively stiff versus wrist flexible) are different. The identical element is hitting an object that is above your head and hitting it down into the ground. This is not a million miles from Judd's theory.

Osgood (1949) developed identical element theory arguing that the key factor is the inter-relationship between the stimuli and responses required. This in turn was further developed by Holding (1976). According to Holding, positive transfer will occur when *a new but similar stimulus requires the use of a well-learned response*. This is called *stimulus generalization*. An example would be a basketball guard who is good at tipping in rebounds and then moves to volleyball. He/she should find setting comparatively easy. However, if a task requires a new and different response to the same or a similar stimulus then negative transfer will occur. This is called *response generalization*. My example of playing a forward defensive shot to the hockey ball is a good example. The ball came to me in a similar way to a cricket ball (it bounced just in front of me) and I responded automatically. I did not do the same when the ball came to me along the ground. This is because the stimulus–response combination was new to me. Holding argued that there would be no transfer either way if both the stimulus and response were completely new.

I am sure that by now you will not be surprised if I said that Holding does not see things as being as simple as that described above. Holding believes that we need to take into account how well learned the task is. The more learned the response, the more likely it is to transfer. This can have major effects on proactive and retroactive transfer. The better a skill is learned the more likely it is to affect the learning of new tasks. However, well-learned responses are less likely to demonstrate retroactive transfer. Many professional cricketers will play golf on their days off. This would appear to be a classic case of risking retroactive inhibition. The fact that their cricket is so well learned means that it is not a problem.

Bilateral transfer

Bilateral transfer, sometimes called *cross-transfer* or *cross-education*, is a special form of transfer. Bilateral transfer refers to *transfer from a limb on one side of the body to another limb on the opposite side of the body, normally the contralateral limb*. Carl Prean, the England table tennis player, was right handed but could play table tennis to county standard with his left hand. Indeed, he sometimes switched hands in a game when trying to get a wide shot to his left-hand side. The tennis player Evgenia Koulikovskaya does this all the time, never playing a backhand. There are many examples of *switch hitters* in baseball, players who can bat left or right handed.

Bilateral transfer does not mean that transfer is easy. What it means is that the person will find acquiring a skill with the non-preferred limb *easier* than if they were learning from scratch. Most athletes, even very gifted ones, still prefer one side to the other, although it may be difficult for most of us to spot. It is also a fact that some very skilful performers have difficulty in using their non-preferred limb even when undertaking lots of practice. The England soccer player Michael Owen is comparatively weak with his left foot, despite a great deal of practice. The great Hungarian footballer of the 1950s, Ferenc Puskas, never used his right foot, it was for standing on only.

There are two theories concerning how bilateral transfer works. The first is that transfer is aided by *knowledge of the principles* involved in the movement. This is very much a cognitivist approach. We know how to perform the skill and so can attempt to control our limbs to bring it about. This is similar to having declarative knowledge, which we need to turn into procedural knowledge. Try some skills for yourself. Choose ones that you do well with your preferred limb. It is thought that the *better a task is learned, with the preferred limb, the better the transfer.*

The second theory came about following EMG research. When a person undertakes physical activity with a limb on the right side of the body, EMG activity is shown to occur in the contralateral limb. It is weak but, nevertheless, exists. This is not really surprising. The left side of the brain controls limbs on the right side of the body and vice versa. However, although the neural pathways cross over in the lower centres of the CNS, there are some ipsilateral pathways. These send neural messages, albeit weak ones, to the limbs on the same side of the body. It is thought that these weak traces mean that the person is not starting from scratch when learning with the opposite limb. Physiotherapists have made use of this fact when treating injured athletes. If the athlete uses the contralateral uninjured limb there is some transfer of strength to the injured limb. It does not totally stop muscle wastage but limits it. Similarly, although we see disparities in the measurements between the preferred and non-preferred arms of tennis players or legs of soccer players the differences are difficult to spot with the naked eye.

Feedback

In Chapter 7, we looked at how proprioceptive feedback aids movement. In Figure 1.4, this is represented by the bottom feedback loop, from output back to input. In this section, we examine feedback as a source for aiding learning. In Figure 1.4, this is represented by the top feedback loop, from output to memory. Feedback is the term we use to describe *information resulting from an action or response.* This can be *visual, proprioceptive, vestibular or auditory.* In most cases a movement will result in more than one of these senses providing feedback. If we kick a ball we not only see where it has gone, we also receive proprioceptive feedback telling us what it felt like. While trying to balance on a beam the gymnast receives visual, proprioceptive and vestibular feedback. In striking games, like cricket and baseball, we even hear the sound that the ball makes on the bat, as well as seeing where it went and feeling the movement.

You will often hear commentators saying 'that hit the "sweet spot"'. They know that the ball hit the middle of the bat because of the sound.

This feedback can be *intrinsic* or *extrinsic*. Intrinsic feedback is sometimes called *inherent* feedback. It is available to the performer without outside help. We can see the results of our actions without anyone needing to tell us what happened. The feel of a movement is intrinsic by definition. Extrinsic feedback is information that is provided for us by some 'foreign' body. Extrinsic feedback is also known as *augmented* feedback. The most common 'foreign body' that supplies feedback is the coach. We will examine, in detail, the ways in which coaches do this later in this section.

There are two major forms of feedback, *Knowledge of Results (KR)* and *Knowledge of Performance (KP)*. KR is post-response information concerning the *outcome* of the action. The most obvious form of KR is visual. We see the end product of our action. In some cases, however, we need outside help to be able to make sense of our actions. A long jumper needs to have the distance he/she jumped measured in order to have KR. Similarly, track athletes may need to know the time that they ran. KP, on the other hand, consists of post-response information concerning the *nature of the movement*. The most obvious type of KP is the 'feel' of the movement or, to be more technical, knowledge of the sensory consequences. KP can and does come in other forms, however. We can see videos of our performance. As we have already said we might hear the sound of ball on bat or racket. We can also use biomechanical methods of providing KP, e.g., measuring force, using specially designed platforms (called force platforms). Table 9.1 shows a list of different types of feedback which are available to us.

Table 9.1   Types of feedback

Verbal descriptive	qualitative, e.g., 'too far', 'spot on', 'nearly'
	quantitative, e.g., 'a metre too long', '11.2 s'
Verbal prescriptive	instructions
Motivational	e.g., 'good', 'well done', 'keep trying'
Visual descriptive	demonstration
	video or film
	computer print out, e.g., results of biomechanical analyses
Proprioceptive	feel of the movement
Auditory	e.g., sound of bat–ball contact

Feedback is used in practice primarily to aid learning. Until very recently, it was claimed that learning was not possible without the use of conscious feedback. As we saw in the last chapter, this is not necessarily the case. We can learn implicitly. This raises the question of how we use feedback in a non-conscious manner. There would appear to be no reason why we should not develop neural pathways even if we are not conscious of doing so, as long as we carry out some form of repetitious practice. It may be that conscious use of feedback merely speeds up learning.

Feedback, however, can be used to aid learning indirectly by providing *motivation*. Success and/or failure can inspire us to strive for a better performance. The former Manchester City and Middlesbrough manager Malcolm Allison, in his excellent book *Soccer for Thinkers* (Allison, 1967), tells of how he used extrinsic KR to help one of his players regain his confidence. The player, a gifted international, had lost confidence, which was affecting his performances. He was not, however, playing as badly as he thought. The player, who was normally very creative, had begun to simply play safe. His excuse for this was that his passing had deteriorated. Allison, therefore, had one of the coaching staff count the number of successful and unsuccessful passes the player made and work out his success rate. When the player saw that it was over 80 per cent, he was reassured and went on to play his normal game.

Timing and precision of feedback

Feedback is a form of instruction, but it is instruction during practice and following the athlete's own attempts at performing the skill. As a result the timing of feedback is important. One of the main factors is when to provide feedback following the learners' performance. This is called the *feedback-delay*, sometimes *KR-delay* or *KP-delay* are used. Research has shown that the length of the feedback-delay is of little importance in learning *but* any interpolated activity, activity between performance and the presentation of the feedback, can inhibit learning. We examined this in Chapter 6, when looking at memory. In some situations, it is not possible to eliminate interpolated activity, e.g., during a game of netball the coach must wait until half-time before he/she can give feedback.

Perhaps more important than the feedback-delay is the *post feedback-delay*. This is also sometimes called the *post KR-delay* or the *post KP-delay*. This is *the time interval between the presentation of the feedback and the learner producing the next response*. As with the feedback-delay, interpolated activity will affect learning. The most important factor, however, is the length of the delay. If the time period is *too short*, the learner does not have time to create a new response. As we saw when looking at memory, it takes time to learn. The whole period between trials is called the *inter-trial interval* (see Figure 9.4).

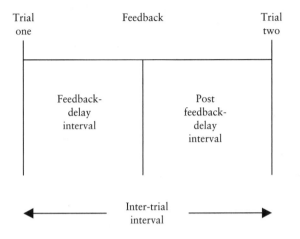

Figure 9.4 Feedback-delay intervals

Another aspect of the timing of feedback is the *frequency* of giving feedback. When talking about frequency of feedback, we use the terms *absolute frequency* and *relative frequency*. Absolute frequency refers to the *total number of feedback presentations* received by the learner. While relative frequency is the *percentage of trials* in which feedback is given. Common sense would say that the higher the relative frequency the better. Surely 100 per cent relative frequency, i.e., feedback following every trial, is best. Research has failed to support this. One of the problems with feedback every trial is that the athlete becomes dependent on the coach. It should be the aim of the coach to get the athlete to be able to use intrinsic feedback and not have to depend on extrinsic feedback. This, however, is not the only factor affecting the efficiency of feedback nor is it the most important. There are other factors that determine which type of feedback is the most beneficial.

One of the first areas to be researched was *precision* of feedback. Just how precise does feedback need to be? At one extreme, we have the method preferred by Star Trek's Mr Spock, 'you missed by 0.46782 cm recurring, Captain'. At the other end is the type of feedback used by comedian Harry Enfield, 'you didn't want to do that'. Neither of these are of much use. The first method is too detailed and as a result it ends up being meaningless. Even giving information which may appear to be easy to understand might also be of limited use. If you are told you were '1 m too long', would you know how far that is? Try it: draw a line 1 m long, without using a ruler or tape measure, then measure it. How near were you? This should be comparatively easy and you should not have been too far away, but how far is 90 cm, 1.25 m and so on?

The Harry Enfield method tells us nothing that we cannot see for ourselves. You may think that no-one would use such a method, but many years of examining and coaching on Football Association award courses has shown me that they do. What we need is something in between. There is an *optimal* level for each *task* and *performer*. Some tasks require more precision than others, if we are to get them right. A dressage rider needs to be 'spot on', whereas a hurdles jockey does not require the same precision when getting over the hurdles. The nature of the learner or performer is also very important. I had the privilege of sitting in while Peter Keen, former Technical Director of the British Cycling team, was giving feedback to a number of different cyclists. To most he gave feedback about intensity, duration and frequency of training in non-scientific language. However when giving feedback to the former Olympic gold medallist, Chris Boardman, he used language and concepts with which most third-year Sports Science undergraduates would have difficulty. Judging by Boardman's questions he was more than capable of handling this level of feedback.

The level of knowledge of the performer is not the only factor, with regard to the learner, that must be taken into account. Research has shown that beginners and experienced performers require different amounts of feedback. Beginners generally require a comparatively large amount of extrinsic feedback, with a fairly high relative frequency. As they develop their expertise, however, they need less and less extrinsic feedback. Therefore, the use of what we call the *fading technique* is recommended. In other words, feedback is given less and less often as the athlete improves. Ideally there will come a time when extrinsic feedback is no longer required. As the old cliché says 'good coaches make themselves redundant'.

Not only should the frequency of feedback alter as the performer improves but so should the type of feedback. In the early stages of learning, the athlete requires not only KR but also KP. They need the KP to develop new movement patterns. At this stage they are not able to do this for themselves, as their knowledge base is poor. They need what we call *prescriptive* feedback. They need to be told what to do in order to improve performance. As they improve and increase their knowledge of the activity, all they require is KR. If they are making an error, they can resolve the problem themselves. So we say that they now require *descriptive* feedback.

Recent research into feedback has examined what is termed *bandwidth* feedback. This kind of feedback developed due to problems with the precision of feedback. As we have seen, feedback can be too precise, thus making it redundant. In Chapter 7, we saw that it is not possible to repeat motor skills precisely every time. The amount of degrees of freedom that must be controlled means that even the great performers cannot be 100 per cent accurate all of the time. Bandwidth feedback takes this into account. The coach sets parameters for performance. If performance falls outside the parameters, feedback is given. If the performer is within the parameters or bandwidth, nothing is said. This kind of feedback has generally, although not unequivocally, been seen to be the most beneficial. It should be remembered that by using bandwidths the coach is, in fact, giving feedback after every trial. If the coach says nothing, the learner knows that they were within the bandwidth, which is a form of KR.

Another issue which concerns the giving of feedback is whether it should be *positive* or *negative*. Positive feedback can be telling someone that he or she has done well. It can also be what we call *constructive* feedback, i.e., the coach tells the learner how to improve performance by saying, 'do it this way'. Negative feedback concentrates on errors. Sometimes coaches point out errors and then follow up with constructive feedback. Constructive feedback has been shown to be effective following either a negative or positive approach. However, negative feedback often includes 'don't do it like that' or 'you got it wrong – you did this and shouldn't have'. This latter type of feedback can be very demotivating and is also of little use to beginners, as they need constructive, prescriptive information. Experienced performers, with large egos, may be able to handle the extreme of negative feedback but I would not recommend trying it unless you know the performer very well indeed.

Before leaving feedback, I should point out that most of the research into feedback has been laboratory based and has used tasks that have little ecological validity with regard to acquiring sports skills. A fair amount of recent research has attempted to use ecologically valid tasks. In real-life situations, there is nearly always some form of feedback available to the performer. KR is present in most tasks. We can normally see what the outcome is, e.g., if I fire an arrow at a target I can see where it struck, or if I shoot in netball, I can see where the ball went – did I score, hit the rim or miss altogether? As we saw with Malcolm Allison's footballer, however, this may not always be the case in team games. KR is not always obvious. This can be because there is too much interpolated activity. It can, also, be because the player thinks that something is good when in fact it is not. In Chapter 2, we talked about my centre-forward who passed to the right-midfield player when he should have passed to the left-midfield player. Had I not pointed this out to him, he would have thought that he had been successful because the ball went where he wanted.

Dynamical Systems Theory and pratice

As we saw in the last chapter, the Dynamical Systems model of instruction is to *set the goal* for the learner and to utilize *constraints* to achieve that goal. Newell (1986) said that when planning a practice we should take into account all three constraints – task, environmental and organismic. Newell claimed that the three have a triangular effect on learning (see Figure 9.5). Practice should take into account this interaction.

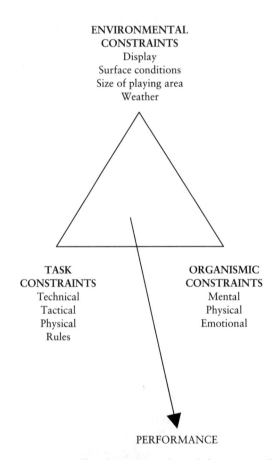

Figure 9.5 How constraints affect learning (adapted from Newell, 1986); reproduced with kind permission of Kluwer Academic Publishers

A number of years ago, I observed an experienced teacher teaching the set shot in basketball to a group of 12-year olds. They used a full-size basketball court, with the basket at the normal height of 3 m (10 ft) and full-size basketballs. Many of the children were less than 1.6 m (5 ft 4 in) tall. There was no way in which they were going to be able to score from even close to the basket never mind from the free throw line. Some managed to get the ball somewhere near the basket by throwing two handed. These he chastised for not using the correct technique. In reality, there was no correct technique for these children for this task. The task and environmental constraints did not match the organismic constraints. Another example of this is children aged 8 and 9 years playing 11-a-side hockey or soccer or 15-a-side Rugby Union, often on full-size pitches. They do not have the physical abilities to play in this environment. Moreover, their stage of cognitive development and lack of experience means that they are weak in selective attention. Both the English Rugby Football Union and The Football Association have recognized this and insist on children playing on smaller pitches, with smaller goals and with less players per side. This inter-action between constraints and practice is not limited to children. When teaching basketball to a group of first-year university students who were beginners, I was exasperated by the fact that they bunched together. When I managed to get them to utilize the whole width of the court, I had a problem in that, because of poor technique, they were unable to pass the ball the distances required.

Being aware of the three-way interaction between task, environmental and organismic constraints allows the coach to manipulate one, two or all three in order to provide the kind of practice that will result in the desired effect. For example, most coaches and teachers, when introducing Rugby for the first time, allow the learners to pass the ball forward. Once they are satisfied that the group is becoming comfortable handling the ball, they impose the task constraint that the ball must be passed backwards. They will probably ban tackling in the beginning. Touch or tag Rugby will be played followed by the introduction of proper tackling. So the task constraints are altered. This is an example of how task constraints can be changed to help develop the practice so that eventually the learners can play a game of Rugby within the laws of the game.

Altering task constraints can also be used to develop specific skills. If a hockey coach wants to help his/her players to utilize the full width of the pitch they can make a rule that goals can only be scored from a pass from the wing. Basketball coaches, who want to develop passing skills, might not allow players to dribble with the ball. Altering the rules in this way is using what we call *conditioned games*. Conditioned games do not only mean using task constraints. Environmental constraints can also be used. Tennis coaches who wish to develop their players' backhands might play a cross-court game – from backhand court to backhand court. Badminton coaches often use narrow long courts, if they want to develop overhead clears.

The manipulation of task and environmental constraints is a common practice in sport, although I doubt that coaches use the word constraint. Manipulating organismic constraints is less common. Practising while tired is a form of organismic constraint and may be very important in some activities. There is good evidence that, when we are tired, we alter the way in which we perform skills. You simply have to watch a tired person performing a skill. Often they are successful but the dynamics of the performance are different from normal. They appear laboured and lack smoothness.

In the last chapter, we looked briefly at the notion of freezing and unfreezing degrees of freedom. This, of course, takes place during practice. In the early stages the coach should set constraints that force the learner to freeze the degrees of freedom. As the performer becomes better, the coach can get the learner to release some degrees of freedom. When teaching the backhand in table tennis the coach will begin with a simple push, with no backspin. To do this the learner must control the degrees of freedom around the wrist, in other words keep the wrist locked. The coach will then ask the player to put backspin on the ball or hit a target, which cannot be achieved unless backspin is added. Backspin requires the player to make contact with the ball using a sweeping motion, which brushes underneath the ball on contact. This can only be achieved by unfreezing the degrees of freedom around the wrist.

Manipulating constraints can also help with selective attention and decision making or, in ecological psychology terms, attunement to affordances. A practice that I use a great deal in soccer is to play six-a-side on a very small pitch. This means that the players are in a shooting position most of the time but have very little time before being tackled. They soon learn that they must look to shoot as quickly as possible. This leads them to recognize the affordance of shooting. The problem with this is will they still look for that affordance when the constraints are taken off? The Dynamical Systems theorists claim that they will, but will also be aware of other affordances.

Practical implications

Of all of the topics covered in this book, practice is the most important. Without practice no learning will take place. We are all aware of the cliché 'practice makes perfect'. In fact, this is incorrect. It is truer to say, *'practice makes permanent'*. If we practise incorrect techniques these will become automatic and are then difficult to change. Sometimes performers think that they have eradicated bad habits only to find themselves returning to them when under pressure. Therefore, it is important that practice is carried out correctly.

In the last chapter, we examined the factors that we must take into account before deciding what the athlete should learn and how the coach should instruct the athlete. In deciding how to practice very similar factors must be taken into account. The type and length of practice that is optimal will be affected by the motivation of the learners. Tiger Woods is happy to undertake long repetitious practice. He is highly motivated and the rewards are great. Many amateur golfers become bored easily with repetitions, so need to constantly change tasks and maybe even have some form of game within the practice. The age of the learner is also important. The younger they are the more active they need to be. Young children will not sit and listen; they need to be playing. Older people, on the other hand, like to have things explained to them in some detail. Children under 11 years are less concerned with competition than those over 11 years. They will take part in cooperative practices, while those over 11 years prefer competition.

The weather too is a factor. It is fine for Brazilians to practise ball juggling on the beach at Copacabana in the height of summer. It is not appropriate in Blackpool in the middle of winter. In this latter case, the players should be kept active and massed practice may well be best. The problem can be the opposite, i.e., too much heat can mean that the coach should adopt spaced practice, allowing plenty of breaks for rest and drinks. Whether to use whole or part-progressive practice will depend on the type of task and the abilities and skills of the learners. If the task is not too exacting, with regard to decision-making and/or neuropsychological components, whole practice is the better. However, if the learners are limited in ability, part-progressive practice may be better.

Time is also a major concern. We have seen that contextual interference aids learning. It is not possible, however, to always use contextual interference if we have little time to spend practising. We may need to determine which is the most important skill and work at that. *Time spent practising* is more important than considerations like contextual interference, type of feedback and whether it is whole or part, massed or spaced practice. Table 9.2 gives a list of considerations which coaches should use in determining what type of practice to use.

Once the coach has decided what type of practice to use, he/she must *organize* the learners, environment and equipment effectively. Getting the environment right is crucial. Earlier, we examined the problems facing a class of 12-year olds playing the set shot in basketball on a full-size court. The environment should have been changed for them. They could have stood nearer to the basket, used a smaller ball and a lower ring. The area in which the performers must work is important. Area is a constraint and as such can affect learning. The area can be too large for the learner, e.g., 10-year olds playing tennis on a full-size court. Nor should it be too small. They need space and time

Table 9.2 Factors affecting choice of type of practice

Learners	Task	Coach/teacher
Motivational level	Cognitive demands	Skills
Cognitive development	Motor demands	Abilities
Motor development	Physical demands	Past experience
Physical development	Safety factors	
Skills		
Abilities		
Fitness levels		

in which to perform. Beginners, at hockey, often have trouble controlling the ball – it takes them time and space. Therefore, they need a larger area when practising than more experienced players, who can control the ball with their first touch.

Also, facilities must be used correctly. I recently watched a student teacher giving a basketball lesson. He was teaching the lay-up. There were six basketball rings in the sports hall but he used only one. Thus, there was a great deal of standing around. Precious practice time was wasted. This is not an unusual happening nor is it confined to trainee teachers and coaches. Table 9.3 lists a number of the considerations that should be taken into account when deciding how to organize a practice session.

Table 9.3 Factors affecting practice organization

Facilities	Environment
Types of learning areas available	Size of learning areas available
Equipment available	Weather conditions
Safety	Learners
Is equipment safe?	Numbers
Is environment safe?	Self discipline
Are spotters/supporters needed?	Age

Once the practice is under way, the coach needs to decide when to give feedback, what kind of feedback to give and when to progress (sometimes it is necessary to regress to more basic skills) in order to move the learner on from what he/she can already do (bootstrapping). This is very easy to say. It is also very easy *theoretically* to know the answers to these problems. It is far more difficult in reality. I have seen many coaches constantly looking at their watches. They have decided, before starting the session, that they will spend 2 min on the first practice, move to practice two, which will take 5 min, then on to practice three and so on. This is totally unrealistic. The amount of time spent practising any task will depend on how well the learners are coping: 5 min may be far too short, it may also be far too long. If they are already capable they may well become bored. This is particularly true with children. The only way to know when and how to move on is by *observation* of the performance. It is also observation that provides the information necessary to provide feedback. We need to know what the performer is doing right and wrong in order to give useful feedback. A trick used by many coaches, who do not fully know what is happening, is to give general feedback to the whole group and simply regurgitate the common faults that they have seen listed in a coaching manual. Good coaches give general feedback *and* feedback to individuals. *Observation is a skill.* It needs to be practised, itself.

Good observation requires selective attention and declarative knowledge. Many coaches go into sessions not knowing enough about the skill which they are coaching. For beginner coaches and teachers, I strongly recommend the use of checklists. Coaches need to be sure that they know the key factors involved in performing the skill. Knowledge of common faults is a help but should be used as an aid to observation not be used instead of observation. Even experienced coaches use checklists but they do not need to write them down – they are 'in their heads'. In Table 9.4, I have given a checklist for heading a

Table 9.4 Checklist for performance of attacking heading in soccer

1. Is the player making contact with the ball using his/her forehead?
2. Is the contact point above the central horizontal axis of the ball?
3. Is the contact point along the central vertical axis?
4. Is the ball headed downwards?
5. Is the upper body arched prior to contact?
6. Does the player 'attack' the ball, i.e., move the upper-body position from being arched to being bent forward, after making contact with the ball?
7. Is the follow through in the line that the player wishes the ball to take?
8. Is the timing of the forward movement of the body correct?

soccer ball. You can test how well you know the basic skills of your own sport by choosing a skill and writing down a list of key points and seeing how that compares with what is written in the coaching manuals.

Once the observations have been made, the coach must determine the type of feedback to be used. Different tasks and performers require different types of feedback. Table 9.5 provides guidelines for determining the type of feedback. Table 9.5 does not take into account whether feedback should be visual, verbal or both. We covered this with regard to instruction but it is equally important with feedback. The same principles apply.

Table 9.5   Factors affecting type of feedback provided

Cognitive development of learner
Emotional development of learner
Personality of learner
Stage of skill acquisition
Motivation of learner
Learner's declarative knowledge of the task
Learner's procedural knowledge of the task
Facilities available to the coach, e.g., videos, computers
Coach's ability to demonstrate

Key points

Information Processing Theory and practice

- Practice can be

    o   massed (intervals between trials are less than the time it takes to do one trial) or spaced (intervals between trials are greater than the time it takes to do one trial),

    o   whole (practising the whole skill): part (practising part of the skill in isolation of the other parts): part-progressive (practising one part of the skill, then adding another part and so on),

    o   whole–part–whole practice (practising the whole then breaking it down into parts and then returning to the whole).

- According to Schema Theory, practice should follow the principle of variability:

  o variability of practice means practising with different initial conditions, this requires different response parameters and, therefore, aids error labelling,

  o research with children has shown that variability of practice results in better retention than using the same initial conditions.

- Random (practising two or more skills with random trials on the different skills) and serial (practising more than one skill in a serial order) practice produce better retention than blocked (practising one skill continuously without interference from the practice of other skills) practice – this is called the contextual interference effect:

  o Shea and Morgan claim that this is because random and serial practice 'force' the learner to develop more strategies to help perform the skill,

  o Lee and Magill believe that it is because each time the person returns to a skill they must reconstruct their action plan,

  o blocked practice produces better performance than random and serial, i.e., performance over the final set of practice trials is better than that shown by those following random or serial practice.

- The contextual interference effect is not shown if the skills are simply variations of the same generalized motor program.

- Transfer of training refers to the effect of the practice of one task on the performance or learning of another task:

  o transfer can be positive (aids performance) or negative (inhibits performance),

  o proactive facilitation is when the practice of a task aids the performance of a subsequent task,

  o proactive inhibition is when the practice of a task negatively affects the performance of a subsequent task,

- ○ retroactive facilitation is when the practice of a new task aids the performance of a previously learned task,

- ○ retroactive inhibition is when the practice of a new task negatively affects the performance of a previously learned task.

- Intra-task transfer of training is when practising one variation of a skill aids or inhibits the performance of a different variation.

- The main theories of transfer of training are:

  - ○ general elements theory (positive transfer occurs when tasks require the same or similar general principles and/or neurological pathways),

  - ○ identical elements theory (positive transfer will occur if the purpose of the responses required are similar),

  - ○ stimulus generalization (positive transfer occurs when a new but similar stimulus requires the use of a well-learned response),

  - ○ response generalization (negative transfer will occur when a familiar stimulus requires a new and different response).

- Bilateral transfer of training is transfer from using a contralateral limb; this is thought to occur because:

  - ○ we can use the same general principles to perform the skill, and/or

  - ○ because ipsilateral neural pathways mean that the contralateral limb has already experienced some learning.

- Feedback is all information resulting from an action.

- Feedback can be intrinsic (from within the person themselves) or extrinsic (from an outside body).

- Feedback can be Knowledge of Results, KR (information concerning the outcome of the action) or Knowledge of Performance, KP (information concerning the nature of the movement).

- The feedback delay (the time between performing the skill and receiving feedback) can be negatively affected by interpolated activity (activity taking place during the delay).

- The post-feedback delay (the time between receiving feedback and having another try) can be negatively affected by interpolated activity:

  o if the post-feedback delay is too short, the learner does not have time to reconstruct their action plan.

- Too much feedback can lead to the learner becoming coach dependent:

  o beginners need a lot of feedback, this should be slowly reduced as the person learns the skill – this is called the fading technique.

- Feedback needs to be meaningful to the learners:

  o very detailed precise feedback can be too difficult for the learner to understand,

  o very limited imprecise feedback can mean nothing to the learner,

  o beginners need prescriptive feedback (they need to be told what they did wrong and how to put it right),

  o experienced performers need descriptive feedback (they need to be told the outcome).

- The use of bandwidth feedback can aid learning:

  o feedback is only given if the response falls outside of parameters (the bandwidth) set by the coach.

Dynamical Systems Theory and practice

- The coach sets the goals.

- In order to achieve the goals, the coach imposes constraints on the practice:

- task constraints limit rules (i.e., use of conditioned games, e.g., in soccer you can only score with a header),

- environmental constraints limit the area to be used (e.g., practising hockey on a small pitch to 'force' players to use the full width),

- organismic constraints can be used to get players to practise in problematic situations (e.g., playing while fatigued).

- Degrees of freedom should be frozen early in practice and released (unfrozen) as the individual learns the skill.

Test your knowledge

(Answers in Appendix 3.)

Part one

Choose which of the phrases, (a), (b), (c) or (d), best completes the statement or answers the question. There is only *one* correct answer for each problem.

1. Skills that are not too difficult technically and tactically are best learned using:

    (a) whole practice,

    (b) part practice,

    (c) part-progressive practice,

    (d) whole–part–whole practice.

2. Skills that are high in information processing demands are normally best learned using:

    (a) whole practice,

    (b) part practice,

    (c) part-progressive practice,

    (d) whole–part–whole practice.

3. Skills that are high in neurophysiological demands are normally best learned using:

  (a) whole practice,

  (b) part practice,

  (c) part-progressive practice,

  (d) whole—part—whole practice.

4. When learning complex skills to be used in a game that is unfamiliar to the learner, it is best to use:

  (a) whole practice,

  (b) part practice,

  (c) part-progressive practice,

  (d) whole—part—whole practice.

5. An experienced athlete trying to eradicate a technical problem would be best advised to use:

  (a) whole practice,

  (b) part practice,

  (c) part-progressive practice,

  (d) whole—part—whole practice.

6. Fatigue is most likely to be a problem when using:

  (a) massed practice,

  (b) spaced practice,

  (c) variable practice,

  (d) blocked practice.

7. Reactive inhibition (boredom) is most likely to be a problem when using:

   (a) massed practice,

   (b) spaced practice,

   (c) variable practice,

   (d) serial practice.

8. According to Schema Theory, the only way that we can build up recall and recognition schemas is to use:

   (a) massed practice,

   (b) spaced practice,

   (c) variable practice,

   (d) serial practice.

9. In skill learning, blocked practice trials are said to lead to:

   (a) good performance but poor retention,

   (b) good performance and good retention,

   (c) poor performance but good retention,

   (d) poor performance and poor retention.

10. In skill learning, serial practice trials are said to lead to:

   (a) good performance but poor retention,

   (b) good performance and good retention,

   (c) poor performance but good retention,

   (d) poor performance and poor retention.

11. According to Shea and Morgan (1979), the contextual interference effect occurs:

   (a) due to variability of practice,

   (b) because it forces the learner to use more strategies to carry out the skill,

(c) because the learner needs to reconstruct the action plan each time they go back to a skill,

(d) because it lessens the reactive inhibition effect.

12. In which of the following situations would you expect a soccer goalkeeper to be most affected by positive transfer of training?

(a) making a dig in volleyball,

(b) catching a rebound in basketball,

(c) making a catch in cricket,

(d) serving in tennis.

13. In which of the following situations would you expect a soccer goalkeeper to be most affected by negative transfer of training?

(a) making a dig in volleyball,

(b) catching a rebound in basketball,

(c) making a catch in cricket,

(d) serving in tennis.

14. An experienced performer, having difficulty in learning a new sport, may be being affected by:

(a) retroactive facilitation,

(b) retroactive inhibition,

(c) proactive facilitation,

(d) proactive inhibition.

15. Playing hockey may help an inexperienced soccer player with his/her positional play. This is an example of:

(a) retroactive facilitation,

(b) retroactive inhibition,

(c) proactive facilitation,

(d) proactive inhibition.

16. Intra-class transfer of training refers to:

    (a) transfer due to the ageing process,

    (b) transfer between two different tasks,

    (c) transfer between different variations of the same task,

    (d) transfer between different sports.

17. According to Judd (1908), positive transfer in decision making between playing soccer and hockey would occur because:

    (a) they have similar general principles,

    (b) they have similar neuropsychological pathways,

    (c) they contain identical elements,

    (d) motivation will be high because of the similarities.

18. According to Holding (1976), a cricketer using a baseball catcher's glove for the first time, would experience negative transfer because:

    (a) a baseball has a different texture to a cricket ball,

    (b) he/she has to use their non-preferred hand,

    (c) the stimulus is the same but the response is different,

    (d) the stimulus is different but the response is similar.

19. According to Holding (1976), which of the following would result in positive transfer:

    (a) kicking a soccer ball and kicking a Rugby ball,

    (b) batting in baseball and batting in cricket,

    (c) serving in tennis and in badminton,

    (d) doing the long jump and the high jump.

20. An experienced basketball player should learn the set shot with their non-preferred hand faster than someone with no experience of basketball because:

    (a) they know the general principles of playing the shot,

(b) they will be more motivated,

(c) they are used to using their non-preferred hand for other skills,

(d) they know the court dimensions.

Part two

Below are a number of questions (Q) and answers (A). Fill in the spaces using the phrases below.

1. Q. What name is given to _____?

    A. Feedback.

2. Q. What is the name for feedback that is _____?

    A. Intrinsic feedback.

3. Q. What is the term used to describe _____?

    A. Extrinsic or augmented feedback.

4. Q. What name do we give to _____?

    A. Knowledge of Results.

5. Q. What name do we give to _____?

    A. Knowledge of Performance.

6. Q. What do we call _____?

    A. The feedback delay period.

7. Q. What do we call _____?

    A. The post-feedback delay period.

8. Q. What do we call the _____?

    A. Relative frequency of feedback.

9. Q. What kind of feedback should _____?

    A. Prescriptive.

10. Q. What kind of feedback should _____?

    A. Descriptive.

11. Q. What name is given to the process whereby as an athlete's expertise increases he/she is _____?

    A. The fading technique.

12. Q. What is the process of giving feedback only _____ called?

    A. Bandwidth feedback.

percentage of trials in which feedback is given   feedback delay
feedback given by a coach   inter-trial interval
information resulting from an action or response   experts receive
given less and less extrinsic feedback   beginners receive
the time between presentation of feedback and the performer's next response
information concerning the nature of a movement
is available to the performer without outside help
the period between the athlete performing the skill and receiving feedback.
when performance falls outside of chosen parameters
information concerning the outcome of an action

Part three

Fill in the blank spaces using the phrases below.

1. Playing conditioned games, such as not allowing dribbling in basketball, is a way of using _____ to aid learning.

2. Playing hockey on a small pitch forces the players to work hard to find space. This is a form of _____.

3. Games like mini-tennis and mini-Rugby were designed in order to take into account the _____ of the learners.

4. Telling someone who has become proficient at the forehand drive in tennis, to play a topspin drive forces them to _____.

5. A learner who is having trouble co-ordinating their movements needs to _____.

6. When learning, young children like _____ before receiving instruction.

7. When learning, older adults like _____ before starting to practice.

8. Practising in bad weather does not affect learning but can _____.

9. Good coaches make sure that their equipment is organized and that the learners are placed _____

10. In deciding how and when to progress from one practice to another coaches need to _____ with the present practice.

11. To aid observation coaches should_____.

environmental constraint   in suitable environment
try the skill for themselves   unfreeze the degrees of freedom
freeze the degrees of freedom   observe how well the learners are coping
organismic constraints   affect motivation
task constraints   use checklists
to receive as much information as possible

Additional reading

Barrett KR (1979) Observation of movement for teachers – a synthesis and applications. *Motor Skills: Theory into Practice* 3: 67–76

Cox R (1999) Psychological considerations of effective coaching. In: *The coaching process*, Cross N and Lyle J (Eds). Butterworth Heinemann, Oxford, UK, pp. 67–90

Franks I (1977) Technique and skill improvement in conditioned games. *Coach* 3: 21–25

Knudson DV and Morrison CS (2002) Intervention: strategies for improving performance. In: *Qualitative analysis of human movement*, Knudson DV (Ed). Human Kinetics, Champaign, Illinois, USA, pp. 127–146; 221–240

10 Arousal and Performance

Learning Objectives

By the end of this chapter, you should be able to

♦ define arousal

♦ understand the major theories of arousal, including

◊ Yerkes–Dodson's Theory

◊ Easterbrook's cue utilization theory

◊ Drive Theory

◊ Kahneman's allocateable resources theory

♦ understand the practical implications for coaches and performers

Acquisition and Performance of Sports Skills   T. McMorris
© 2004 John Wiley & Sons, Ltd   ISBNs: 0-470-84994-0 (HB); 0-470-84995-9 (PB)

Introduction

Modern textbooks on motor learning and performance rarely cover the effect of arousal on performance. It is normally left to writers covering social psychology or sports psychology. The motor learning authors of the 1960s, such as Cratty (1967), Oxendine (1968) and Singer (1968), looked upon the arousal–performance interaction as being part of their domain. Social and sports psychologists rarely cover the effect of arousal on skill acquisition. Indeed, when examining the arousal–performance interaction, they focus on the former often paying little attention to the latter. As a result, I felt that I should include the topic in this book. It, also, helps to bridge a gap between the study of sports psychology and motor behaviour. This gap has developed over the years as psychologists have specialized more and more. This has become so acute that, in many British Universities, sports psychology is studied but not skill acquisition and performance, despite the obvious inter-relationship.

The terms arousal and anxiety are often confused in the sports science literature. Anxiety can be a cause of changes in arousal but it is not arousal. Moreover, anxiety is not the only cause of changes in arousal. Increases in arousal are seen when individuals get excited, while decreases are observed when they become despondent. *Arousal is induced by changes in emotions.* Any kind of emotion will affect arousal. This, however, does not tell us what arousal is. There does not appear to be any universally recognized definition of arousal. This is probably one of the reasons for it becoming confused with anxiety. Based on reading many definitions, I will proffer the working definition that *arousal is the physiological and/or cognitive readiness to act.* This definition is somewhat different from some of the early theories, which concentrated on physiological factors. These are often termed unidimensional theories. It also differs from some of the later ideas, such as those of Pribram and McGuinness (1975) and Sanders (1983), which differentiate between the readiness to act and the readiness to respond. The definition which we are using is closest to that of Humphreys and Revelle (1984), who defined arousal as a *'peripheral somatic or physiological response to a situation and/ or biochemical central response to a situation'*. The 'biochemical central response' is what I have termed 'cognitive readiness'. These later theories of arousal all accept that it is both a peripheral (physiological) and central (within the CNS) phenomenon. We will examine that claim later in this chapter.

Inverted-U theories

Yerkes–Dodson Theory

The first researchers to examine the effect of arousal on performance were Yerkes and Dodson in 1908. Yerkes and Dodson tested the ability of mice to negotiate a maze while under different amounts of a stress (electric shocks). The stress was to increase arousal from baseline – no shock at all. They found that when arousal was low, performance was poor. As arousal rose, it reached an optimal level and performance was better. If arousal continued to rise, however, performance deteriorated until it eventually returned to a level equal to that shown during low levels of arousal. When plotted graphically, performance demonstrated an inverted-U curve (see Figure 10.1). Yerkes and Dodson's theory of arousal became known as *inverted-U theory* and is still the most widely accepted arousal–performance theory.

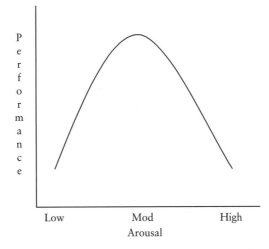

Figure 10.1 Yerkes and Dodson's inverted-U model of the arousal–performance interaction (based on Yerkes and Dodson, 1908)

Yerkes and Dodson continued their experimentation and tested how complexity of the task would affect the inverted-U curve. They found that if a task were easy, the curve was skewed towards the higher end of the arousal continuum, while if the task was complex, it was skewed the other way (see Figure 10.2). In other words, *easy tasks require high levels of arousal* for optimal performance, while *complex tasks require lower levels of arousal*. The beauty of Yerkes and Dodson's theory (often simply referred to as the *Yerkes–Dodson Law*) is its

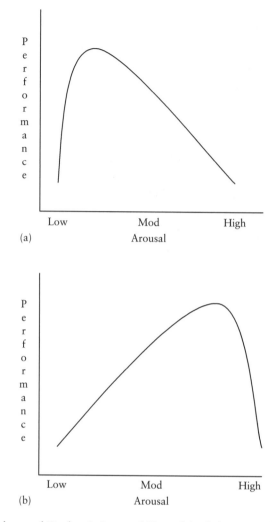

Figure 10.2 Yerkes and Dodson's inverted-U model of the arousal–performance interaction when tasks are (a) simple or (b) complex (based on Yerkes and Dodson, 1908)

intuitive appeal. We can easily see this in action, particularly in sport. End of the season basketball games, between middle of the league teams, often demonstrate the effect of low levels of arousal. The players have little to play for and 'just go through the motions'. In play-off games, however, they can be too aroused, with the same effect – performance is poor. In important, but not vital, games we often see optimal performance. We can also see the effects of task complexity. Chess players, while producing optimal performance, are low in arousal compared with boxers. We can even see this in team games like Rugby and American Football. Different players will require different levels of arousal to produce optimal performance, depending on their position. The quarterback does not want to be as aroused as the linemen or the scrum half as the prop forwards.

Easterbrook's cue utilization theory

Although Yerkes and Dodson's theory was, and still is, widely acclaimed it was criticized for failing to explain why and how arousal affects performance. As a result Easterbrook developed *cue utilization theory*. According to Easterbrook, when arousal level is low people attend to *too many cues and attend to irrelevant as well as relevant cues*. As arousal rises, attention reaches an optimal level, when only relevant cues are processed. This corresponds to the top of the curve in Yerkes and Dodson's theory. If arousal continues to rise, however, attention will narrow and even relevant cues will be missed, hence deterioration in performance with high levels of arousal. Figure 10.3 provides a diagrammatic explanation of this.

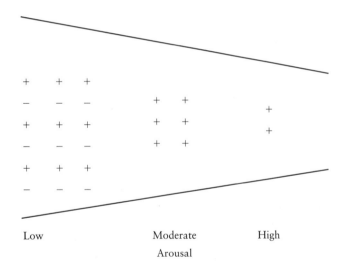

Figure 10.3 Diagrammatic description of Easterbrook's cue utilization theory (from Landers, 1980); reprinted with permission from *Research Quarterly for Exercise and Sport*, Vol. 51, 77–90, 1980 by the American Alliance for Health, Physical Education, Recreation and Dance, 1900 Association Drive, Reston, VA 20191, USA

Although this theory is also still widely accepted, I must admit to having some problems with it. I do not think that it has the intuitive appeal of Yerkes and Dodson's theory. I am far from convinced that, when we are at low levels of arousal, we attend to too many cues. I do not accept that we are likely to attend to irrelevant cues at the expense of relevant ones. My own experience of playing sport when under-aroused is that my problem was attending to too few cues, relevant or irrelevant. Something similar to what we saw with Signal Detection Theory, errors of omission. Also, at high levels of arousal, I believe that the problem is not an over-narrowing of attention but rather attention becoming focused on irrelevant cues. This is especially so when we are over-aroused due to anxiety. We begin to focus on the causes of our anxiety rather than on the task at hand. We will return to these points when examining allocateable resources theories later in this chapter.

Drive Theory

An alternative to inverted-U theories was put forward by Hull (1943), and later developed by Spence (1958). It is called *Drive Theory*. Drive Theory developed from Hull's observation that high levels of arousal do not always result in a deterioration in performance. They do sometimes but not always. Similarly, moderate levels of arousal do not always result in optimal performance. Indeed in some cases arousal has no effect on performance whatsoever. I personally accept these claims made by Hull. Do you? Think about your own performances. Have you always reacted in an inverted-U manner or have there been disparities, as Hull claimed?

According to Drive Theory, increases in arousal will result in an increase in performance, *if habit strength is high*. If *habit strength is low* then increases in arousal will either have no effect or will result in a breakdown in performance. Hull and Spence claimed that the equation is further complicated by the *incentive* value of completing the task. They stated that there would be an *interaction between arousal, habit strength and incentive value*. This interaction could be explained by the formula

$$P = D \times H \times I$$

where P is performance, D is drive or arousal, H is habit strength and I is incentive value. By 'habit strength' Hull and Spence mean *how well learned a skill is*. If their theory is correct, this has a major impact on the arousal–learning inter-relationship. If high levels of arousal were likely to lead to a breakdown in performance, it would be foolish to have beginners practise while in a high-arousal state. On the other hand, experienced performers will produce optimal performance only when highly aroused. We often see players looking good in practice games but 'falling apart' when placed in a real game. Similarly, there are good examples of high arousal leading to optimal performance. When there is pressure some athletes 'raise their game', to use a cliché. We even talk about some athletes as being 'big-game players' – the bigger the competition the better they play. This latter factor is what Hull and Spence mean by incentive value, *how important the activity is to the performer.* This will particularly have an effect on drive or arousal.

Drive Theory is often depicted graphically by a straight line (see Figure 10.4). This is incorrect. A straight line will only be demonstrated if the task is well learned. If not, it may act as in Figure 10.5. Drive Theory is in many ways the 'forgotten theory' of arousal and performance. There are some interesting factors about it, however. Hull and Spence recognized that arousal is more complex than a simple uni-dimensional response.

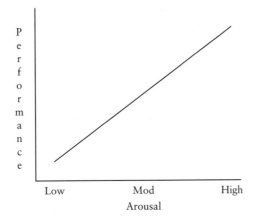

Figure 10.4 Drive theory: arousal–performance interaction when habit strength is high

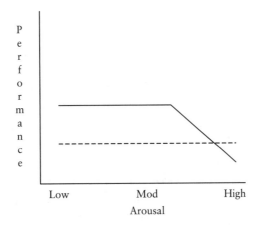

Figure 10.5 Drive theory: arousal–performance interaction when habit strength is low (NB there are two possibilities)

Allocateable Resources Theories

The notion that arousal is not uni-dimensional has been developed by theorists proposing *allocateable resources* theories. The first of these theories was put forward by Kahneman (1973). Kahneman believes that individuals have limited amounts of resources. The amount is not fixed but flexible. Kahneman claims that as arousal rises the number of resources available, within the CNS, increases. Like Yerkes and Dodson, he argues that this increase is beneficial for performance up to a certain point, after which there will be a return to base levels of performance. It is here that Kahneman disagrees with Yerkes and Dodson. To Kahneman increase in arousal is not the only factor affecting performance. The increase in the number of resources, as arousal increases to a moderate level, will only result in improvements in performance if the person *allocates* the resources to the task in hand.

The allocation of resources to task relevant information is said to be undertaken by *cognitive effort* (often just referred to as *effort*). Kahneman believes that performance, even at low levels of arousal, can be optimal if cognitive effort allocates resources to task relevant information. This can be seen when we perform well because we are composed and not emotionally aroused. Similarly, Kahneman does not see high levels of arousal leading to a narrowing of attention. Rather, he sees the problem as not being able to allocate resources to the task. For example, the person starts to focus on their feelings of distress or excitement. You may well have experienced both of these emotions. If anxiety is causing over-arousal, we begin to think what others may think if we fail. Or, in adventure education tasks, we may begin to concentrate on the possibility of injury. On the other hand, one often sees tennis players performing well against someone who is expected to beat them. They suddenly realize that they can, and will, win if they continue to play this well. They then begin focusing on the winning rather than on the task at hand and end up losing.

Kahneman believes that, at high levels of arousal, cognitive effort cannot overcome the emotional factors and so is unable to allocate resources effectively. Michael Eysenck (1992) has challenged this and claims that, even when arousal is high, cognitive effort can allocate resources to the task if the skill is well learned. The best example ever given to me to support Eysenck came in one of my Master's degree classes. One of the students had been a member of the Special Air Service (SAS). I asked him if he had ever been shot at, I assume that this is very arousing indeed (I hope that the experience will remain an assumption). He answered that he had. When I asked how the arousal had affected him, he stated that he became totally focused on the task and responded as he had done in the many hours of practice he had undertaken, ready for such an event.

The notion that resources increase with arousal is not based on some whim of Kahneman. There is evidence to show that as arousal rises there are increases in CNS concentrations of *nor-adrenaline* (sometimes called *nor-epinephrine*) and *dopamine*. Nor-adrenaline and dopamine are neurotransmitters, which play large roles in the person's readiness to respond and act.

Practical implications

Changes in arousal levels have implications for the performance and acquisition of skills. We have already stated that beginners have difficulty in performing when under high levels of arousal. This has major implications for the type of practice that coaches might use. Anxiety and excitement need to be controlled as much as possible. The more complex the skill the less the arousal, if learning is to be optimal. This is not always as simple as it appears. When I was a physical education teacher, I often had to teach students immediately after they had had a mathematic lesson. When they arrived at PE, they were very excited. This meant that I had to calm them down before trying to teach them anything. On other occasions, especially first lesson in the morning, it was necessary to increase arousal before trying to teach anything.

As individuals begin to become more competent, they need to be exposed to a greater level of arousal. It is of little use if the skills can only be performed under no pressure at all. Top-class performers must be able to play even when very highly aroused. This can be even more important in the military, as we saw earlier with my SAS student.

Warm-up decrement

Alterations in arousal during practice can also affect the performance curve. This happens due to the phenomenon known as *warm-up decrement* (WUD). It is well documented, with non-sports activities, that performance following a period of rest will show a temporary decrease – this is WUD. After a few trials, performance will return to the level it was at when practice was interrupted (see Figure 10.6). WUD affects performance but not learning. Nacsson and Schmidt (1971) claimed that WUD was the result of the person losing concentration or changing their *activity set*. Activity set, or psychological set, is what we are

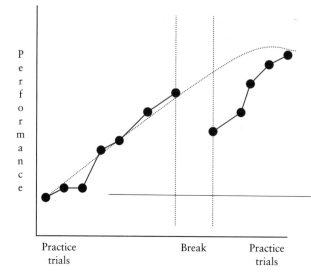

Figure 10.6 Graphical description of warm-up decrement

focusing on. During practice the person is focusing on the task. In other words, cognitive effort is allocating resources effectively. During the rest period, the learner begins to lose concentration and focuses on non-task specific factors. When they resume the activity, it takes time for effort to re-focus the mind to the task.

Anshel and Wrisberg (e.g., 1993) have argued that WUD is simply the result of decreases in physiological arousal. They have provided some evidence for this. Exercise taken, while not practising the task, does appear to reduce or even eliminate WUD. WUD is not only a factor with beginners. In sports like basketball and ice hockey, where there are many substitutions, the WUD effect is often demonstrated when a player returns to the game. It often looks as though the player is 'lost' and the game is 'going on around them'. Some players try to maintain the correct activity set by following the game closely or by using imagery to ensure that arousal is optimal. The Manchester United manager, Sir Alex Ferguson, claims that Ole Gunnar Scholksjaër is a good player to send on as a substitute because, when he is on the bench, he follows the game very closely unlike many other players.

Warm-up

If moderate levels of arousal are beneficial for performance, it would appear that using a warm-up would aid performance. Very little research has examined the effect of warm-up on the performance of skills. What research there has been suggests that warm-up has a positive effect. However, the intensity of exercise needed is quite surprising. Research, including my own, has shown that exercise needs to be at least 60 per cent of maximum intensity. This is far higher than most sports performers would undertake.

What needs to be examined is whether a general warm-up (physical activity only) is as useful as a task specific warm-up (physical activity plus performing the skill). The latter would appear to be the better as it combines increases in nor-adrenaline and dopamine with helping the person to acquire the correct activity set. I first came across this type of warm-up when coaching soccer in Canada. On returning to Britain, I used it with some success. Moreover, the players felt that it was beneficial.

Just as there has been little research into the effect of warm-up on performance, there has been very little examining the effect of heavy and fatiguing exercise on the performance of sports skills. Exercise physiologists have looked at running and swimming, while fatigued, but few have examined the effect of exercise on skills that require perception and decision making as well as motor control. What little research there has been suggests that fatigue does not affect learning. It probably affects performance but it is difficult to say whether this is due to a direct effect of exercise or perception of discomfort. When the exercise is for the specific limbs which are controlling the movement being performed, e.g., a volleyball player repeatedly jumping to make blocks, then it is definitely a direct effect. The depletion of neurotransmitters results in a loss of co-ordination and power. However, if the exercise is general, e.g., running then having to read a map as in orienteering, it would appear that perception of fatigue, rather than a direct effect of exercise, is the cause of poor performance. Another example of this would be a hockey player doing a great deal of running and then having to shoot at goal.

Key points

- Arousal is the physiological and/or cognitive readiness to act.

Theories of arousal–performance interaction

- Yerkes–Dodson's inverted-U theory:

- o   low and high levels of arousal induce poor performance,

- o   moderate levels of arousal lead to optimal performance,

- o   complex skills require lower levels of arousal than simple skills, for optimal performance.

- Easterbrook's cue utilization theory:

  - o   an inverted-U theory,

  - o   at low levels of arousal, attention is focused on relevant and irrelevant information,

  - o   at moderate level of arousal, attention is on relevant cues only,

  - o   at high levels of arousal, attention narrows to focus on relevant cues but not all of them.

- Drive theory:

  - o   performance is dependent on the interaction between drive (arousal), habit strength and incentive value of performing well,

  - o   if habit and incentive are high, the greater the arousal and the better the performance,

  - o   if habit and/or incentive are low, increases in arousal will either have no effect on performance or lead to a breakdown.

- Kahneman's allocateable resources theories:

  - o   an inverted-U theory,

  - o   as arousal increases so do the number of resources available to the individual,

  - o   at low arousal, performance will be poor unless cognitive effort can allocate sufficient resources to the task,

- o at moderate arousal, performance will be optimal if cognitive effort allocates resources to the task,

- o at high levels of arousal, it is difficult for cognitive effort to overcome the negative effects of too many resources, therefore performance will be poor.

Practical implications

- Use warm-up to make sure that arousal is optimal.

- Task specific warm-up may be better than a general warm-up, as the activity set hypothesis suggests that this type of warm-up helps the athletes focus on the task.

- Exercise can eliminate the warm-up decrement effect.

Test your knowledge

(Answers in Appendix 3.)

Part one

Fill in the blank spaces using the phrases below.

1. Arousal is induced by _____.

2. Arousal is the _____ readiness to act.

3. Pribram and McGuinness (1975) differentiated between the readiness to act and _____.

4. According to Yerkes and Dodson (1908), moderate levels of arousal should _____.

5. A weight lifter would be expected, by Yerkes and Dodson (1908), to require _____ for optimal performance to be demonstrated.

6. A chess player would be expected, by Yerkes and Dodson (1908), to require _____ for optimal performance to be demonstrated.

7. According to Easterbrook (1959), as arousal increases _____.

8. Easterbrook (1959) would expect someone performing in an unimportant game _____.

9. At high levels of arousal, Easterbrook (1959) believes that we miss relevant cues because _____.

10. According to Drive Theory, performance at high levels of arousal will be better than at low and moderate levels if _____.

11. In their formula, Hull and Spence used the term _____ to denote the importance of the activity.

12. Kahneman (1973) stated that, as arousal increases, _____.

13. Kahneman (1973) believes that performance under low levels of arousal can be as good as when arousal is moderate as long as _____.

14. When arousal increases there are also_____ nor-adrenaline and dopamine.

15. Warm-up decrement is observed when there is a temporary decrease in performance _____.

16. Nacsson and Schmidt (1971) claimed that warm-up decrement occurs because during rest we change our activity set or, in other words, we _____.

comparatively high levels of arousal
so does the amount of allocateable resources
readiness to respond
following a period of rest:
increases in the neurotransmitters
to attend to irrelevant cues
comparatively low levels of arousal
cognitive effort allocates sufficient resources to the task
focus on information that has nothing to do with the task

attention narrows too much
attention narrows
habit strength is high
physiological and or cognitive
induce optimal performance
changes in emotions
incentive value

Part two

Which of the following statements are true (T) and which are false (F)?

1. Humphreys and Revelle (1984) believe that arousal is
   peripheral only.   T   F

2. According to Yerkes and Dodson (1908), American Football
   quarterbacks would require different levels of arousal from
   100 m sprinters if optimal performance were to be shown.   T   F

3. According to Easterbrook (1959), at low levels of arousal
   we attend to irrelevant as well as relevant cues.   T   F

4. According to Drive Theory, if habit strength is low
   performance may not be affected by changes in arousal.   T   F

5. According to Drive Theory, if habit strength is low
   performance may deteriorate as arousal increases.   T   F

6. Eysenck (1992) believes that, even if arousal is high, optimal
   performance can occur if a task is well learned and
   cognitive effort allocates resources to the task.   T   F

7. Kahneman (1973) and Easterbrook (1959) agree that with
   a high level of arousal there is a narrowing of attention.   T   F

8. When arousal rises, there is an increase of nor-adrenaline
   in the CNS.   T   F

9. Anshel and Wrisberg (1993) showed that exercise alone
   could not reduce the effect of warm-up decrement.   T   F

10. Fatigue does not affect performance.   T   F

Additional reading

Wrisberg CA (1984) Stress and performance. *Motor Skills: Theory into Practice* 7: 47–55

11 Conclusion

Introduction

In this chapter we will examine, firstly, the 'state of the art' – what we know about skill acquisition and performance – and then the position of the paradigm battle between Information Processing Theory and ecological psychology theories. The 'state of the art' includes some facts for which we have little or no explanation, either from a cognitive or ecological perspective. Hopefully, this will give you some ideas for future research which will be of interest to you. Some of you will need to undertake research projects as part of your degree programme, while others may simply wish to carry out research to try to find out what really is happening with regard to a phenomenon that is of interest to them.

State of the art

Observation of human beings performing sports skills shows clearly that we have a vast array of such skills. Some of these skills could be more correctly described as being techniques, i.e., motor acts requiring little in the way of perception or decision making. Other skills have a large working memory component. Many skills are carried out very quickly. Today, cricket and baseball batters must hit balls projected at over 180 km/hr (100 mph). Similarly, gymnastic skills which were once considered to be outstanding are now commonplace. To win a medal in top-class gymnastics, the performer has to demonstrate movements which require exceptionally good co-ordination and must, also, be aesthetically pleasing. In the rest of this section, we will examine what is agreed upon by sports psychologists, regardless of which school of thought they are in, with regard to these skills.

Acquisition and Performance of Sports Skills   T. McMorris
© 2004 John Wiley & Sons, Ltd   ISBNs: 0-470-84994-0 (HB); 0-470-84995-9 (PB)

Skill

In Chapter 1, we examined the nature of skill and its classification. There appears to be no contradiction to the notion that skill is learnt and consistent. Although not all sports psychologists like the use of classifications, examination of the literature in this field shows that the terms open and closed skill, discrete, serial and continuous skill; and complex and simple skill are commonly in use. Open skill is mostly used to describe skills in which perception, decision making and/or anticipation play a major part; the term closed skill is used to describe actions which are more concerned with technique than information processing.

The notion of discrete, serial and continuous skill is self-evident but has implications when considered alongside skill acquisition. It is the complex–simple classification which appears to cause the major concern. Some authors stick rigidly to the idea that simple skills have little input from information processing, while complex skills rely heavily on this factor. Thus the terms are used synonymously with closed and open skills. Other authors include the co-ordination or neuropsychological demands when classifying skills as being simple or complex. For example, the task of chipping a golf ball out of a bunker onto the green is hardly a simple skill, yet it would be classed as such by those authors who ignore the neuropsychological factors. A small, but growing, band of authors prefers to use factor analysis to describe the nature of skills rather than to classify them. It appears to me that this approach could be beneficial, especially when trying to decide how to teach a skill.

Abilities

The case with abilities is far less straightforward. It is very unusual today to see authors refer to abilities *per se*. Ecological psychologists use the term organismic constraints, while developmental psychologists refer to mental, physical and neuropsychological limitations. Even exercise physiologists are aware of factors limiting performance. In sports psychology, however, it appears to be unfashionable to talk about abilities. Indeed, Anders Ericsson and his followers argue that the idea that abilities limit possible levels of achievement is incorrect and that with practice we can all acquire any skill we wish. The arguments put forward by Ericsson are out of the scope of an introductory text like this one but should be of interest to you as you develop your knowledge. Despite the claims of Ericsson, the notion that we have underlying abilities which determine our potential has intuitive appeal.

Perception

The area of perception is arguably the most controversial with regard consensus of agreement among sports psychologists. However, some factors *are* considered to be indisputable. Everyone accepts the importance of perception in skilled performance. The key factor in open skills would appear to be selective attention. Whether we believe selective attention comes about as a result of building up a memory bank or whether it is because of attunement to affordances, the indisputable fact is that it is important. It is also generally agreed that visual perception is more important than other types, not only to aid information processing but also to control movement. This is not to say that other types of perception are redundant. Similarly, the interaction between perception and action is seen to be a major factor in deciding what to do and actually carrying out the action.

Decision making

The area of decision making is one which has received little in the way of research. That there are individual differences in peoples' ability to make decisions is not disputed but we have very little idea why there are differences. It is appearing more and more that such differences are due to task specific factors rather than underlying abilities. Nevertheless, there is still a large group of sports psychologists who believes that there are underlying factors but we have simply been unable to isolate them. This is an area which requires much more research.

Reaction time

The consensus of opinion with regard to reaction time is that humans can perform very quickly but there *are* time constraints. This is demonstrated both in the laboratory and in real-life situations. It is also accepted that factors such as complexity of the display, type of stimulus and nature of the response affect reaction time. In more recent times, it has become generally accepted that an individual's reaction time in a sports-specific situation may be very different from that measured in a laboratory. Also, a short reaction time in one activity does not appear to mean that the person will have a short reaction time in another activity. This is a large move away from the ideas of the 1960s, when both the Americans and the Soviets thought that testing reaction times in laboratories could help them to identify potential champion athletes.

Anticipation

The need to utilize perceptual anticipation, especially in fast ball games, is also generally accepted. More sophisticated technology has allowed us to research this phenomenon in recent years. Few would argue that it does not occur. It is also agreed that learning to anticipate may well take place at a sub-conscious level rather than be learnt explicitly. As with decision making, however, why and how individuals differ remains difficult to determine.

Motor control

With regard to motor control, it is agreed that both the CNS and PNS play crucial roles in ensuring that movement is accurate and controlled. The importance of the role of visual proprioception is a new area which has become generally accepted, as is the idea that action commands are general rather than specific, with the PNS playing a refining role.

Memory

Little is fully agreed upon about memory, except that it is used to determine goals for action. If we accept that 'attunement to affordances' is another way of saying 'memory' then it could be argued that there is agreement that some form of rehearsal is necessary for memory to be developed. It would also appear that there are limitations to the capacity of short-term memory and to the time it takes to develop a representation in the CNS.

Learning

The fact that coaches and teachers can aid learning is accepted by both Information Processing theorists and ecological psychologists. Similarly, the effect of maturation, physical and mental, is readily accepted by both schools. It is also accepted that some form of feedback is necessary for learning to take place but this may take place at a sub-conscious level. As a result, it is now believed that learning can be implicit. As stated concerning memory, the need for some form of rehearsal is also universally recognized as being essential. A much neglected area, both in research and theoretically, is the use and abuse of instruction and demonstration. These areas require much more research.

Practice

Practice is almost certainly the least controversial area in skill acquisition. Practice is essential for learning to take place. On many occasions I have had individuals come to me and ask how they can get better at a particular task. When I tell them to practice, practice and practice again, they think that I cannot be bothered with them. The reality, however, is that there is no secret. Practice is the key.

Information Processing Theory versus ecological psychology theories

Perhaps of more interest than areas in which sports psychologist agree are those areas in which they disagree. Before examining these differences we should remind ourselves that while the two schools differ in their explanations of some factors, in many they are simply trying to explain the same phenomena but from different perspectives. Information Processing Theory is primarily concerned with the role of the CNS in skill acquisition and performance. On the other hand, the ecological psychologists are more interested in overt behaviour and try to explain skill without reference to the CNS, because we do not know what is happening there. They are interested in what we see directly rather than what we infer from what we see. The latter is the domain of the Information Processing theorists. This fundamental difference is probably highlighted best in beliefs about perception.

To the Information Processing theorists perception takes place in the CNS and requires the interpretation of sensory information based on past experience. It is dependent on memory. The ecological psychologists see perception as being direct – taking place in the periphery with no recourse to memory. To Information Processing theorists perception precedes action, while the ecological psychologists believe that perception and action are coupled – they are both responsible for perception and are both responsible for action. Although this is somewhat confusing it is, in fact, of little difference from what the Information

Processing theorists are saying. The ecological psychologists argue that in order to perceive we must act – even if this action is just scanning the display. Similarly, when we move we use feedback from the afferent nerves to control the action, therefore action is not separate from perception. This to a large extent is semantics. Moreover, it does not disagree fundamentally with the Information Processing theorists, who accept that we must search the environment for cues and accept that sensory feedback aids movement.

Interceptive actions, also, highlight the difference between the two schools. To the cognitivists, interceptive actions can only take place because we compare the present situation to past experiences stored in memory. To the ecologists, the optic array, present in the environment, supplies all of the necessary information in the form of τ. No past experience is necessary.

Similarly, with regard to selective attention the Information Processing theorists see it as depending on experience, while to the ecological psychologists it is merely searching the display for affordances and is dependent on the goals that the action requires. The ecologists see this as an answer to how we achieve our goals, while the cognitivists see decision making as being the end product of working memory.

The explanation for the whole nature of skill acquisition also differs between the two schools. To the cognitivists, it is all about developing memory representations, while to the ecologists the aim is to help the individual become attuned to the affordances in the environment. The former is thought to be acquired by explicit *and* implicit learning, while the latter is the result of the organization of constraints and is, therefore, implicit in nature. The individual is not told 'do it like this', as the Information Processing theorists would suggest, but is told 'when performing this task you must obey these rules'. These constraints then 'force' the learner to produce the required action.

This brings us to one of the major areas of difference between the two schools. To the Information Processing theorists action is controlled by the CNS. The PNS may play a very minor role and fine tune a movement but it is the CNS that is crucial. To the ecological psychologists the CNS simply sets the goals. The movement is under the control of the PNS.

The challenge for sports psychologist at the moment is to come to some consensus of opinion with regard to what is the best explanation of how we perform skills. There are obviously 'die-hard' supporters of each of the schools who will never alter their opinion. However, many sports psychologists are moving towards a hybrid theory. As we have seen throughout this book, each theory has its strengths and weaknesses, and each explains one aspect better than another. Undoubtedly areas such as decision making and reaction time are best explained by the Information Processing theorists, while movement may be better explained by the ecologists. More thought and research is necessary before coming to a conclusion. This should serve as a warning to you that you are studying a 'living' science where the answers, and even the questions, are constantly changing. You need to be aware that we are a long way from knowing, for certain, how we acquire and perform sports skills.

Writing an Academic Paper

Appendix 1

Immediately below is a version (version one) of an extract from an unpublished paper, McMorris, T., Sproule, J. and MacGillivary, W. W. (2000) 'Field Dependence/Independence, Gender and Motivation of Kinesiology Students for Participation in Sport', written in the same style as I have used in this book. This is followed by the original (version two), written in the style recommended by the *American Psychological Association (APA)*. Note in particular that, in the *APA* version, *all* statements referring to theory and previous research include a citation of the original work.

Version one

A great deal of research has examined the relationship between Field Dependence (FD)/Field Independence (FI) and sport performance or the effect of FD/FI on the performance of sport. Authors have generally argued that FI individuals would have an advantage over FD in the sporting arena because FI individuals can disembed figures from their background, solve problems analytically, have the ability to cognitively reconstruct a display and can articulate visuo-vestibular cues. FD persons, on the other hand, have relative difficulty in disembedding objects from their background, solve problems intuitively, are dominated by the existing display and have difficulty in articulating visuo-vestibular information.

Witkin called this aspect of his FD/FI theory perceptual style. However, he further developed his theory to include other aspects of cognitive functioning. The present study is concerned with what Witkin termed a 'sense of separate identity'. Witkin claimed that FI individuals use internal frames of reference when making decisions and can detach themselves from environmental influences. FD people, however, are reliant on external sources when making decisions.

Acquisition and Performance of Sports Skills   T. McMorris
© 2004 John Wiley & Sons, Ltd   ISBNs: 0-470-84994-0 (HB); 0-470-84995-9 (PB)

This difference between FD and FI persons has led some researchers to hypothesize that FD individuals will prefer to perform in team sports while FI people will choose individual activities. There is some evidence to support this hypothesis but it is by no means unequivocal. I believe that the unequivocal nature of the results is due to the fact that, while it is reasonable to expect FD individuals to choose team sports because of their reliance on external sources of reference, FI individuals would be equally at ease in both team and individual activities. In the team situation FI persons can perform as part of the team but their goals for taking part and their evaluation of their performance will be self referenced rather than team referenced. Following this line of thinking, while it may be too simplistic to compare the FD/FI of team and individual sports performers, it is possible that FD and FI persons differ in the type of motivation for participation in sport, regardless of whether it is team or individual activities.

Factor Analysis has consistently identified competition and affiliation as key components of motivation. Affiliation has been defined as the desire to participate in order to interact with others. There is some disagreement about exactly what is meant by competitive motivation, however. Roberts (1984) argued that there are two forms of competition motivation. One of these he terms competitive motivation, which he claims is characterized by an emphasis on social comparison – the desire to win or to perform well in comparison to others. The other he terms mastery, which is characterized by the intrinsic desire to perform to the best of one's ability regardless of the outcome.

Version two

A large amount of research has been undertaken into Field Dependence (FD)/ Field Independence (FI) and sport (see MacGillivary, 1980; McMorris, 1992 for reviews). Almost all of this research has examined the relationship between FD/FI and sport performance or the effect of FD/FI on the performance of sport. The same can be said of more recent research (e.g., McMorris *et al.*, 1993; McMorris, 1997; Tenenbaum *et al.*, 1993). Authors have generally argued that FI individuals would have an advantage over FD in the sporting arena because FI individuals can disembed figures from their background, solve problems analytically, have the ability to cognitively reconstruct a display and can articulate visuo-vestibular cues. FD persons, on the other hand, have relative difficulty in disembedding objects from their background, solve problems intuitively, are dominated by the existing display and have difficulty in articulating visuo-vestibular information (Witkin and Goodenough, 1980).

Witkin called this aspect of his FD/FI theory perceptual style (Witkin, 1950). However, he further developed his theory to include other aspects of cognitive functioning. The present study is concerned with what Witkin and associates termed a 'sense of separate identity' (Witkin *et al.*, 1971). Witkin *et al.* claimed that FI individuals use internal frames of reference when making decisions and can detach themselves from environmental influences. FD people, however, are reliant on external sources when making decisions.

This difference between FD and FI persons has led some researchers to hypothesize that FD individuals will prefer to perform in team sports while FI people will choose individual activities. There is some evidence to support this hypothesis but it is by no means unequivocal (see Brady, 1995; McLeod, 1985; McMorris, and Cobb, 1993; Pargman, 1977; Pargman, Schreiber, and Stein, 1974). McMorris and Cobb claimed that the unequivocal nature of the results was due to the fact that, while it is reasonable to expect FD individuals to choose team sports because of their reliance on external sources of reference, FI individuals would be equally at ease in both team and individual activities. In the team situation FI persons can perform as part of the team but their goals for taking part and their evaluation of their performance will be self referenced rather than team referenced. Following this line of thinking, while it may be too simplistic to compare the FD/FI of team and individual sports performers, it is possible that FD and FI persons differ in the type of motivation for participation in sport, regardless of whether it is team or individual activities.

Many Factor Analytical studies have examined reasons why people take part in sport and many factors have been determined (e.g., Ashford, Biddle and Goudas, 1993; Buonamano, Cei and Mussino, 1995; Gill, 1988; Gill *et al.*, 1996; White and Duda, 1994). Two factors that are consistently identified are competition and affiliation. Affiliation has been defined as the desire to participate in order to interact with others (McMorris and Cobb, 1993) and there appears to be little variation in what different authors perceive as comprising affiliation. Competition motivation, however, is more difficult to define.

Taking a theoretical stance, Roberts (1984), basing his ideas on Nicholls' (1984) theory of achievement motivation, has argued that there are two forms of competition motivation. One of these he terms competitive motivation, which he claims is characterized by an emphasis on social comparison – the desire to win or to perform well in comparison to others. The other he terms mastery, which is characterized by the intrinsic desire to perform to the best of one's ability regardless of the outcome.

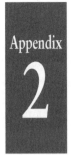

Appendix 2

Glossary of Terms Used by Ecological Psychologists

The terms marked * are not used in this book, although what they explain is covered.

affordances   opportunities for action – what the environment allows us to do.

attunement to affordances   becoming aware of where, in the environment, affordances are most likely to occur.

constraints   factors which limit an action, or 'force' the individual to behave in a specific way.

control parameter*   any factor which causes the person to alter their order parameter (see environmental, organismic and task constraints).

co-ordinative structures*   the muscles, joints and nerves which self-organize to control movement (see self-organization).

degrees of freedom   the muscles, joints and nerves which need to be controlled when making a movement.

direct perception   meaningful perceptual information, present within the environment, which does not require interpretation.

disequilibrium*   period when control parameters lead to a phase transition (see phase transition).

environmental constraints   constraints imposed by the environment, e.g., weather conditions.

equilibrium*   period when there is no desire or need to alter the order parameter (see order parameter).

freezing the degrees of freedom   limiting the movement of muscles and joints.

functional specificity instructions from the CNS, which are concerned with the holistic picture of what we wish to do rather than being specific muscle commands.

order parameters*   the way in which a movement is carried out; the nature of the self-organization at that specific moment in time.

organismic constraints   constraints resulting from the individual's physical, mental and emotional strengths and weaknesses, e.g., height.

perception–action coupling   interaction between perception and action in order to act upon the environment; action is necessary for perception to take place and perception is necessary for action to take place.

phase transition*   changing order parameters due to the effect of control parameters.

realization of affordances*   carrying out an action.

Acquisition and Performance of Sports Skills   T. McMorris
© 2004 John Wiley & Sons, Ltd   ISBNs: 0-470-84994-0 (HB); 0-470-84995-9 (PB)

self-organization   limbs interact to affect control of movement.

task constraints   constraints which occur as a direct result of the nature of the task, e.g., rules of a game.

τ **(tau)**   mathematical calculation of the time to contact; the time it takes for an external object to reach the individual or for the individual to reach the object, determined by the rate of change of the dilation of the image of the object on the retina.

$\dot{\tau}$ **(tau dot)**   the same as τ but taking into consideration the acceleration and/or deceleration of the object or person.

τ **margin***   the same as τ except taking into consideration the fact that our calculation is not precise and that as long as we work within a given margin of error we will be successful (often used inter-changeably with τ).

unfreezing the degrees of freedom   allowing a range of movement in muscles and joints.

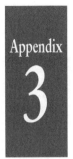

Test Your Knowledge Answers

Appendix 3

Chapter 1

Part one

1. (b), 2. (a), 3. (a), 4. (b), 5. (d), 6. (a), 7. (c), 8. (a), 9. (b), 10. (b), 11. (a), 12. (d).

Part two

1. F, 2. T, 3. F, 4. T, 5. T, 6. T, 7. T, 8. F, 9. F, 10. T, 11. T, 12. T, 13. F, 14. T, 15. F, 16. F, 17. T, 18. F, 19. F, 20. T.

Chapter 2

Part one

1. (b), 2. (d), 3. (b), 4. (b), 5. (a), 6. (a), 7. (c), 8. (d), 9. (a), 10. (c), 11. (a), 12. (b), 13. (d), 14. (c), 15. (c).

Part two

The words added are in *italics*.

1. There are two types of vision, *foveal* and *ambient*.

2. *Audition* can help table tennis players to know the amount of spin that has been placed on the ball.

3. According to Information Processing Theory, *perception* is inferred or *indirect*.

4. According to Information Processing Theory, perception is the organization, *integration* and *interpretation* of sensory *information*.

Acquisition and Performance of Sports Skills   T. McMorris
© 2004 John Wiley & Sons, Ltd   ISBNs: 0-470-84994-0 (HB); 0-470-84995-9 (PB)

5. Swets (1964), in his Signal Detection Theory, stated that detection of a signal would be affected by the *intensity* of the signal compared with the *strength* of the background noise.

6. In Signal Detection Theory, *d*-prime represents the individual's *sensitivity*.

7. In Signal Detection Theory, the criterion represents the individual's *bias*.

8. In tennis, pattern recognition allows us to *anticipate* what shot our opponent is going to play before he/she has hit the ball.

9. When we see an object moving towards us, then lose sight of it, we are still able to 'know' the trajectory of the object because of the phenomenon called *closure*.

10. We need *selective attention* because we are limited in the amount of information with which we can deal at any one time.

11. With regard to CNS capacity, Deutsch and Deutsch (1963) claimed that capacity was *fixed*, while Kahneman (1973) stated that it was *flexible*.

12. According to Kahneman (1973), cognitive effort is responsible for the *allocation* of *resources*.

13. According to Norman (1969), we process information that is *pertinent*.

14. Individuals whose perception of objects is negatively affected by movement are said to be *velocity susceptible*.

15. The amount of information we can perceive in one glance is called the span of *apprehension*.

16. We visually track fast-moving objects using *saccades*.

17. The *intuitive–plastic*–analytic continuum is a theory of perceptual style.

18. According to Action Systems Theory, *action* is necessary for perception to take place.

19. To the ecological psychologists, all the information that we need is present in the display, we do not need *memory*.

20. Ecological psychologists use the term *affordances* to describe what the environment allows us to do.

21. Experience allows us to become *attuned* to affordances.

22. According to Dynamical Systems Theory, information in the environment is *meaningful* and does not have to be processed by the CNS.

Chapter 3

Part one

The words added are in *italics*.

1. Knapp (1963) defined decision making as *knowing which technique to use* in any given situation.

2. Skill consists of *decision making plus technique*.

3. Working memory consists of *perception, decision, short-term memory* and recall from long-term memory.

4. Schemas are *generalized rules*.

5. Declarative knowledge is *knowing what to do*.

6. Procedural knowledge is *knowing what to do and how to do it*.

7. According to Anderson's (1982) ACT Theory, *we predetermine what we will do* in any given situation.

8. Field Independent people *make decisions analytically*.

9. Field Dependent individuals *make decisions intuitively*.

10. According to Dynamical Systems Theory, the CNS *determines the goals to be achieved*.

11. The rules of a game are examples of *task constraints*.

Part two

The words added are in *italics*.

1. To the Information Processing theorists, decision making is determined by our ability to use *perception* and past experience.

2. It is possible to possess a large range of *techniques* and lack skill.

3. Schmidt (1975) claimed that we do not recall specific past experiences but *generalized* rules.

4. Anderson's (1982) ACT Theory explains how we are able to make decisions *quickly*.

5. When learning to make decisions we often follow a *hierarchy* of responses

6. *Declarative* knowledge is supposed to precede *procedural* knowledge, according to Anderson.

7. According to Dynamical Systems Theory, two individuals will interact differently with the same environment because of their differing *organismic* constraints.

8. Weather conditions are an example of *environmental* constraints.

9. Once an affordance to achieve a goal has been perceived, *action* will take place automatically.

10. In research experiments, speed of decisions is measured using a *tachistoscopic* timing device.

11. Helsen and Pauwels' (1988) research design is better than previous designs because the way of measuring the decision is more *realistic*.

12. For the subjective assessment of players' decision making to be effective, the assessors need *guidelines*.

13. Assessors also need to be *experienced*.

14. Research has generally shown that experts make *faster* decisions than novices.

15. Dynamical Systems theorists and Information Processing theorists agree that *experience* helps the person to do make the correct move.

Chapter 4

Part one

The words added are in *italics*.

1. Response time consists of *reaction time and movement time*.

2. Reaction time is the time that elapses from the sudden onset of a stimulus to *the beginning of an overt response*.

3. Reaction time consists of *pre-motor and motor time*.

4. Simple reaction time is when there is only *one stimulus and one response*.

5. 170 to 200 ms represents the *range of mean simple reaction times*.

6. According to the Hick–Hyman Law, as the number of stimuli–response combinations is increased reaction time *increases linearly*.

7. If a stimulus has a 90 per cent probability of being presented, it will demonstrate a reaction time that is shorter than if *it has a 50 per cent chance* of presentation.

8. Dillon, Crassini and Abernethy (1989) claimed that a stimulus with a 90 per cent probability of presentation would be reacted to quickly because we *store responses in a hierarchical order.*

9. Reaction times when the probability of a stimulus being presented is 70 per cent and when it is 50 per cent shows *no significant difference.*

10. The psychological refractory period shows that when two stimuli are presented close together reaction time to the second stimulus will be *longer than normal.*

11. Practice can reduce the psychological refractory period but *cannot eliminate it.*

12. If two stimuli are presented within 50 ms of one another they can *treated as one.*

13. According to Yerkes and Dodson (1908), a moderate level of arousal will induce a reaction time that is shorter than when arousal level is *low or high.*

14. A shorter than normal reaction time will be shown when the stimulus stands out against *the background.*

15. Visual reaction time is longer than *auditory.*

16. If a foreperiod is too short, the person does not have *time to prepare the response.*

17. Complex responses require longer foreperiods because *the response takes longer to prepare.*

Part two

1. F, 2. T, 3. F, 4. T, 5. F, 6. T, 7. F, 8. T, 9. F, 10. T, 11. F, 12. F, 13. T, 14. F, 15. T, 16. F, 17. T, 18. F, 19. F, 20. T.

Chapter 5

Part one

1. (b), 2. (a), 3. (c), 4. (c), 5. (c), 6. (b), 7. (a), 8. (b).

Part two

The words added are in *italics*.

While coincidence anticipation is vital in sports like tennis, *baseball* and *cricket*, perceptual anticipation is very important in team games. Perceptual anticipation refers to the ability of a performer to predict upcoming events based on *partial information.*

There are three main types of perceptual anticipation. *Spatial* is the prediction of where a person thinks an event will occur. *Temporal* anticipation is the timing of an event or when it will happen, while *event* anticipation refers to anticipating what will happen. To the Information Processing theorists, perceptual anticipation is a product of *working memory*. Without past *experience* of similar events, we are not able to anticipate. However, they believe that anticipation can be either *conscious* or *sub-conscious*. Ecological psychologists believe that experience is not essential because all the necessary information is present in the *display*. For example in tennis, information from your opponent's *racket* and *body* are all you need to anticipate what shot he/she is going to play. Anticipation, however, will be aided by the person becoming *attuned to affordances*.

Research into perceptual anticipation originally used a temporal *occlusion* paradigm. Jones and Miles (1978) showed film clips of a tennis player serving to experienced coaches and *inexperienced* tennis players. The film was stopped two frames before *racket–ball contact*, at contact and two frames after. Experienced players were able to anticipate where the ball would land better than the inexperienced players. Jones and Miles measured the difference between where the ball actually landed and where the participant *anticipated*. The amount of error was measured. This is called *radial error*. Jones and Miles' experiment lacked realism because the participants had to mark down on a *map* of the *court* where they thought the ball had landed. Clatworthy, Holder and Graydon (1991) overcame this in a hockey goalkeeping test by having the goalkeepers *simulate* making a save.

Abernethy and Russell (1987) wanted to know what parts of the display provided the most information. Therefore, they *blocked out* parts of the player's body. Research, using eye-mark recorders, has also tried to determine which areas of the display provide the most information. Eye-mark recorders allow the researcher to see what the participant is *focusing on*. Results of this research show that in ball games good players can use *cues* that are present before the ball has been released, in order to decide where it will be going. Most research has measured *expert–novice* differences. As expected, experts have been shown to be superior. Little research has examined *expert–intermediate* differences. Learning studies have shown that *anticipation* can be acquired.

Chapter 6

Part one

1. (a), 2. (d), 3. (d), 4. (b), 5. (b), 6. (a), 7. (d), 8. (d), 9. (d), 10. (a), 11. (b), 12. (a).

Part two

1. T, 2. T, 3. F, 4. F, 5. F, 6. T, 7. T, 8. T, 9. F, 10. F, 11. F, 12. T, 13. F, 14. T.

Chapter 7

Part one

The words added are in *italics*.

1. Q. How did Sherrington (1906) describe *proprioception*?

    A. The perception of the body and its position in space.

2. Q. What does the term *kinesthesis* describe?

    A. The person's perception of the movements of their body and separate body parts.

3. Q. What are the two types of *peripheral vision*?

    A. Horizontal and vertical.

4. Q. To what does the *vestibulo–oculomotor interaction* refer?

    A. The interaction between the oculomotor system and the vestibular apparatus.

5. Q. Which part of the vestibular apparatus is responsible for the perception of the *direction of movement* and changes in acceleration?

    A. Semi-circular canals.

6. Q. Which afferent nerves are situated *between muscles and joints*?

    A. Golgi tendon organs.

7. Q. Which part of the CNS initiates *voluntary movement*?

    A. Pre-motor cortex.

8. Q. Which part of the brain is thought to regulate movements of *less than one reaction time*?

    A. Basal ganglia

9. Q. What is the name given to the process also known as *short-loop feedback*?

    A. α–γ co-activation.

10. Q. Which part of the brain controls movements of greater than one reaction time?

    A. The cerebellum.

11. Q. Which nerves are responsible for passing information from the CNS to the muscles so that *movement can take place*?

    A. Motoneurons or efferent nerves.

12. Q. Which nerves are responsible for passing information *about a movement*?

    A. Sensory or afferent nerves.

13. Q. What did Keele (1968) describe as a *set of muscle commands* that allow movement to be performed without any peripheral feedback?

    A. A motor program.

14. Q. What do Information Processing theorists call the process which allows us to make *minor alterations* to movements in less than one reaction time?

    A. Feedforward.

15. Q. According to ecological psychologists, what is the *role of the CNS*?

    A. To set the goal.

16. Q. What do ecological psychologists mean by *organismic constraints*?

    A. The physical and mental characteristics of the individual, which affect the way in which they carry out a movement.

17. Q. What kind of constraints are *rules of a game*?

    A. Task constraints.

18. Q. How do ecological psychologists describe different *muscles and joints working together*?

    A. Self-organization.

19. Q. What term did Bernstein (1967) use to describe the number of *muscles, joints and nerves* that must be controlled in order to produce a co-ordinated movement?

    A. Degrees of freedom.

20. Q. What name did Lee and Young (1985) give to the time when information from an object results in the *initiation of a movement to intercept*?

    A. (τ) tau.

Part two

The words added are in *italics*.

1. There are two types of peripheral vision, *vertical* and *horizontal*.

2. *Vision* is the most important of the senses with regard to proprioception.

3. We visually track fast movements using *saccades*.

4. The *utricles* and *ventricles* provide information about the position of the head.

5. The *gamma* motoneurons inform the muscle spindles about the tension they should 'feel'.

6. Movements of more than one reaction time are said to be under *closed* loop control.

7. According to Keele (1968), when developing a motor program we firstly form a *template* of the task.

8. Keele (1968) claimed that the development of motor programs takes place in the motor cortex, basal ganglia and *cerebellum*.

9. An Arab spring, flick-flack and somersault, performed as a gymnastics routine, is an example of an *executive* motor program.

10. MacNeilage (1970) believes that we store the *location* of key points in a movement.

11. Schmidt (1975) claimed that we do not store specifics of a motor program but *generalized* rules or schemas.

12. Schmidt's theory explains how we can do the same skill in a *variety* of different ways.

13. Sherrington (1906) asked whether CNS instructions were *muscle* or *movement* commands.

14. According to ecological psychologists, commands from the CNS are *functionally specific*.

15. Two people will perform the same skill differently because they have different *organismic* constraints.

16. A baseball pitcher and a cricket bowler use different actions because of the *task* constraints under which they must perform.

17. Someone doing a somersault in a gymnasium on a sprung floor and then doing the same action on grass will need to alter their movement because of the differing *environmental* constraints.

18. According to ecological psychologists, we do not need to remember a movement because our limbs will carry it out automatically because of *self-organization*.

19. According to Lee and Young (1985), action and perception of the τ margin occur *automatically*.

20. Bootsma and Van Wieringen (1990) used the term *funnel* shape to explain how we control late movement of a bat when striking a ball.

Chapter 8

Part one

The words added are in *italics*

Kerr (1982) defined learning as being a relatively *permanent* change in performance, resulting from *practice* or *experience*. Performance, on the other hand, *fluctuates* from time to time. We cannot directly measure learning, we can only *infer* it based on *performance*. Learning is measured by retention tests. The amount that has been learned is said to be demonstrated by the amount that is retained over a period of *no practice*. Another method of measuring learning is transfer tests. The use of transfer tests is based on the assumption that if a task is well learned it can be performed in *different environments*. The third method commonly used to measure learning is the use of performance *curves*.

When learning some tasks the learner reaches periods when no improvement is shown; these are termed *plateaus*. These periods may be caused by *reactive inhibition*. Learning can be positive or *negative*, but is always demonstrated by *consistency*.

Part two

1. (c), 2. (c), 3. (b), 4. (b), 5. (d), 6. (d), 7. (a), 8. (b).

Part three

The words added are in *italics*.

1.   Q. What do we call a performance curve that demonstrates a great deal of learning in the early stages then *slows down*?

     A. A negatively accelerated curve.

2.   Q. What do we call a *period of no apparent learning*?

     A. A plateau.

3.   Q. What did Anderson (1982) call *knowing what to do*?

     A. Declarative knowledge.

4.   Q. What did Anderson (1982) call *knowing what to do and how to do it*?

     A. Procedural knowledge

5.   Q. What do we call *learning sub-consciously*?

     A. Implicit learning.

6.   Q. What is the most common form of *mental rehearsal*?

     A. Mental imagery.

7.   Q. Which group of psychologists believed that humans learn *by problem solving*?

     A. The Gestältists.

8.   Q. In which phase of learning do Fitts and Posner (1967) claim that we *use verbal labelling*?

     A. Cognitive phase.

9.   Q. According to Gentile (1972), what is developed when the learner is able *to differentiate between relevant and irrelevant cues*?

     A. Selective attention

10. Q. Which of Gentile's (1972) stages of learning is characterized by *fixation and diversification*?

     A. Skill-refinement stage.

11. Q. Which of Adams' (1971) learning stages is similar to Fitts' and Posner's *autonomous stage*?

     A. The motor stage.

12. Q. According to Schmidt (1975), which kind of memory *evaluates the ongoing movement*?

     A. Recognition memory.

13. Q. In developing the recall schema, we remember the *changes in the specifics of the action*. What name did Schmidt (1975) give to this?

    A. Response parameters.

14. Q. Which part of the recognition schema allows us to remember *what the movement feels like*?

    A. Sensory consequences.

15. Q. Why did Schmidt say that it is best to *use variable practice*?

    A. It allows us to experience different initial response parameters and sensory consequences.

16. Q. What does Turvey (1992) say that we should do when learning a new skill in order to control *the movement of muscles and joints*?

    A. Freeze the degrees of freedom.

Part four

1. T, 2. T, 3. F, 4. F, 5. F, 6. F, 7. T, 8. T, 9. T, 10. T, 11. F, 12. T, 13. T, 14. F, 15. F, 16. F.

Chapter 9

Part one

1. (a), 2. (c), 3. (c), 4. (d), 5. (b), 6. (a), 7. (a), 8. (c), 9. (a), 10. (c), 11. (b), 12. (b), 13. (a), 14. (d), 15. (a), 16. (c), 17. (a), 18. (c), 19. (a), 20. (a).

Part two

The words added are in *italics*.

1. Q. What name is given to *information resulting from an action or response*?

   A. Feedback.

2. Q. What is the name for feedback that is *available to the performer without outside help*?

   A. Intrinsic feedback.

3. Q. What is the term used to describe *feedback given by a coach*?

    A. Extrinsic or augmented feedback.

4. Q. What name do we give to *information concerning the outcome of an action*?

    A. Knowledge of Results.

5. What name do we give to *information concerning the nature of a movement*?

    A. Knowledge of Performance.

6. Q. What do we call *the period between the athlete performing the skill and receiving feedback*?

    A. The feedback delay period.

7. Q. What do we call *the time between the presentation of feedback and the performer's next response*?

    A. The post-feedback delay period.

8. Q. What do we call the *percentage of trials in which feedback is given*?

    A. Relative frequency of feedback.

9. Q. What kind of feedback should *experts receive*?

    A. Prescriptive.

10. Q. What kind of feedback should *beginners receive*?

    A. Descriptive.

11. Q. What name is given to the process whereby as an athlete's expertise increases he/she is *given less and less extrinsic feedback*?

    A. The fading technique.

12. Q. What is the process of giving feedback only *when performance falls outside of chosen parameters* called?

    A. Bandwidth feedback.

Part three

The words added are in *italics*.

1. Playing conditioned games, such as not allowing dribbling in basketball, is a way of using *task constraints* to aid learning.

2. Playing hockey on a small pitch forces the players to work hard to find space. This is a form of *environmental constraint*.

3. Games like mini-tennis and mini-Rugby were designed in order to take into account the *organismic constraints* of the learners.

4. Telling someone who has become proficient at the forehand drive in tennis, to play a topspin drive forces them to *unfreeze the degrees of freedom*.

5. A learner who is having trouble co-ordinating their movements needs to *freeze the degrees of freedom*.

6. When learning, young children like *to try the skill for themselves* before receiving instruction.

7. When learning, older adults like *to receive as much information as possible* before starting to practice.

8. Practising in bad weather does not affect learning but can *affect motivation*.

9. Good coaches make sure that their equipment is organized and that the learners are placed *in a suitable environment*.

10. In deciding how and when to progress, from one practice to another, coaches need to *observe how well the learners are coping* with the present practice.

11. To aid observation coaches should *use checklists*.

Chapter 10

Part one

The words added are in *italics*.

1. Arousal is induced by *changes in emotions*.

2. Arousal is the *physiological and/or cognitive* readiness to act.

3. Pribram and McGuinness (1975) differentiated between the readiness to act and *readiness to respond*.

4. According to Yerkes and Dodson (1908), moderate levels of arousal should *induce optimal performance.*

5. A weight lifter would be expected, by Yerkes and Dodson (1908), to require *comparatively high levels of arousal* for optimal performance to be demonstrated.

6. A chess player would be expected, by Yerkes and Dodson (1908), to require *comparatively low levels of arousal* for optimal performance to be demonstrated.

7. According to Easterbrook (1959), as arousal increases *attention narrows.*

8. Easterbrook would expect someone performing in an unimportant game *to attend to irrelevant cues.*

9. At high levels of arousal, Easterbrook (1959) believes that we miss relevant cues because *attention narrows too much.*

10. According to Drive Theory, performance at high levels of arousal will be better than at low and moderate levels if *habit strength is high.*

11. In their formula, Hull and Spence used the term *incentive value* to denote the importance of the activity.

12. Kahneman (1973) stated that as arousal increases *so does the amount of allocate-able resources.*

13. Kahneman (1973) believes that performance under low levels of arousal can be as good as when arousal is moderate as long as *cognitive effort allocates sufficient resources to the task.*

14. When arousal increases there are also *increases in the neurotransmitters* nor-adrenaline and dopamine.

15. Warm-up decrement is observed when there is a temporary decrease in performance *following a period of rest.*

16. Nacsson and Schmidt (1971) claimed that warm-up decrement occurs because during rest we change our activity set or, in other words, we *focus on information that has nothing to do with the task.*

Part two

1. F, 2. T, 3. T, 4. T, 5. T, 6. T, 7. F, 8. T, 9. F, 10. F.

References

Abernethy B (1992) Visual search strategies and decision making in sport. *Int J Sport Psych*, **22**: 189–210

Abernethy B and Russell DG (1987) Expert–novice differences in an applied selective attention task. *J Sport Psych* **9**: 326–345

Adams JA (1971) A closed-loop theory of motor learning. *J Motor Behavior* **3**: 111–149

Alain C and Proteau L (1980) Decision making in sport. In: *Psychology of motor behavior and sport – 1979* Nadeau CH *et al.* (Eds) Human Kinetics, Champaign, Illinois, USA, pp. 465–477

Allard F and Starkes JM (1980) Perception in sport: volleyball. *J Sport Psych* **2**: 22–33

Allard F, Graham S. and Paarsalu ME (1980) Perception in sport: basketball *J Sport Psych* **2**: 14–21

Allison M (1967) *Soccer for thinkers*. Pelham, London, UK

American Psychological Association (2002) *Publication Manual of the APA*, 5th edn. APA, Washington DC, USA

Anderson JR (1982) Acquisition of cognitive skill. *Psych Rev* **89**: 369–406

Anderson, J. R. and Lebiere, C. (1998) *The atomic components of thought*. Lawrence Erlbaum, Hillsdale, New Jersey, USA

Anshel MA and Wrisberg CA (1993) Reducing warm-up decrement in the performance of the tennis serve. *J Sport Exer Psych* **15**: 290–303

Ashford B, Biddle S and Goudas M (1993) Participation in community sports centres: motives and predictors of enjoyment. *J Sports Sci* **11**: 249–256

Baddeley AD (1986) *Working memory*. Oxford University Press, New York, USA

Bandura A (1977) Self-efficacy: toward a unifying theory of behavioral change. *Psych Rev* **84**: 191–215

Battig JW (1979) The flexibility of human memory. In: *Levels of processing in human memory*, Cermak LS and Craik FLM (Eds) Erlbaum, Hillsdale, New Jersey USA pp. 23–44

Bernstein N (1967) *The coordination and regulation of movement*. Pergamon, Oxford, UK

Bootsma RJ and Van Wieringen PCW (1990) Timing an attacking forehand drive in table tennis. *J Exp Psych: Human Perception and Performance* **16**: 21–29

Brady F (1995) Sports skill classification, gender and perceptual style. *Perceptual and Motor Skills* **81**: 611–620

Broadbent DE (1958) *Perception and communication*. Pergamon, Oxford, UK

Bunker D and Thorpe R (1982) The curriculum model. In: *Rethinking games teaching*. Thorpe R, Bunker D and Almond L (Eds) Loughborough University, Loughborough, UK

Acquisition and Performance of Sports Skills   T. McMorris
© 2004 John Wiley & Sons, Ltd   ISBNs: 0-470-84994-0 (HB); 0-470-84995-9 (PB)

Buonamano R, Cei A and Mussino A (1995) Participation motivation in Italian youth sport. *Sport Psych* 9: 265–281

Cherry E . (1953) Some experiments on the recognition of speech with one and two ears. *J Acoust Soc Am* 25, 975–979

Clatworthy R, Holder T and Graydon J (1991) An investigation into the anticipation of field hockey penalty flicks using an ecologically valid temporal occlusion trechnique. *J Sports Sci* 10: 439–440

Cratty BJ (1967) *Movement behavior and motor learning, 1st edn*. Lea and Febiger, Philadelphia, USA

Davids K and Stratford R (1989) Peripheral vision and simple catching: the screen paradigm revisited. *J Sports Sci* 7: 139–152

Deutsch JA and Deutsch D (1963) Attention: some theoretical considerations. *Psych Rev* 70: 80–90

Dewhurst DS (1967) Neuromuscular control system. *IEEE Trans Biomed Eng* 14: 167–171

Dillon JM, Crassini B and Abernethy B (1989) Stimulus uncertainty and response time in a simulated racquet-sport task. *J Hum Move Stud* 17: 115–132

Easterbrook JA (1959) The effect of emotion on cue utilization and the organization of behavior. *Psych Rev* 66: 183–201

Ericsson KA, Krampe RT and Teschromer C (1993) The role of deliberate practice in the acquisition of expert performance. *Psych Rev* 100: 363–406

Eysenck MW (1992) *Anxiety: the cognitive perspective*. Lawrence Erlbaum, Hove, UK

Fitts PM and Posner MI (1967) *Human performance*. Brooks/Cole, Belmont, California, USA

Fleishman EA (1954) Dimensional analysis of psychomotor abilities. *J Exp Psych* 48: 437–454

Fleishman EA (1967) Development of a behavior taxonomy for human tasks: A correlational–experimental approach. *J App Psych* 51: 1–10

Gallahue DL and Ozmun JC (1995) *Understanding motor development*. Brown and Benchmark, Madison, Wisconsin, USA, p. 86

Gentile AM (1972) A working model of skill acquisition with application to teaching. *Quest* 17: 3–23

Gentile AM *et al.* (1975) The structure of motor tasks. *Mouvement*, 7: 11–28

Gibson JJ (1979) *The ecological approach to visual perception*. Houghton Mifflin, Boston, Massachusetts, USA

Gill DL (1988) Gender differences in competitive orientation and sport participation. *Int J Sport Psych* 19: 145–159

Gill DL *et al* (1996) Competitive orientations and motives of adult sport and exercise participants. *J Sport Behavior* 19: 307–318

Glencross DJ and Cibich BJ (1977) Decision analysis of games skills *Australian J Sports Med* 9: 72–75

Goulet C, Bard C and Fleury M (1989) Expertise difference in preparing to return a tennis serve: A visual information processing approach. *J Sport Exer Psych* 11: 382–392

Hale BD (1982) The effects of internal and external imagery on muscular and ocular concomitants. *J Sport Psych*, 4: 379–387

Helsen W and Pauwels JM (1988) The use of a simulator and training of tactical skills in soccer. In: *Science and football*, Reilly T *et al.* (Eds). Spon, London, UK, pp. 493–497

Henry FM (1968) Specificity vs. generality in learning motor skill. In: *Classical studies on physical activity*, Brown RC and Kenyon GS (Eds). Prentice-Hall, Englewood Cliffs, New Jersey, USA, pp. 331–340

Hick WE (1952) On the rate of gain of information. *Quart J Exp Psych* **4**: 11–26

Holder TP (1998) Sources of information in the acquisition and organisation of interceptive actions. Ph.D. thesis, University of Southampton, UK

Holding D (1976) An approximate transfer surface. *J Motor Behavior* **8**: 1–9

Hubbard AW and Seng CN (1954) Visual movements of batters. *Res Quart Exer Sport* **25**: 42–57

Hull CL (1943) *Principles of behavior.* Appleton-Century-Crofts, New York, USA

Humphreys MS and Revelle W (1984) Personality, motivation and performance: a theory of the relationship between individual differences and information processing. *Psych Rev* **91**: 153–184

Hyman R (1953) Stimulus information as a determinant of reaction time. *J Exp Psych* **45**: 188–196

Jones CM and Miles TR (1978) Use of advance cues in predicting the flight of a lawn tennis ball. *J Hum Move Stud* **4**: 231–235

Judd CH (1908) The relation of special training to general intelligence. *Educ Rev* **36**: 28–42

Kahneman D (1973) *Attention and effort.* Prentice-Hall, Englewood Cliffs, New Jersey, USA

Keele SW (1968) Movement control in skilled motor performance. *Psych Bull* **70**: 387–403

Kerr R (1982) *Psychomotor learning.* Saunders, Philadelphia, USA. p. 5

Knapp B (1963) *Skill in sport: the attainment of proficiency.* Routledge and Kegan Paul, London, UK, p. 3

Kroll W and Clarkson PM (1978) Fractionated reflex time, resisted and unresisted fractionated time under normal and fatigued conditions. In: *Psychology of motor behavior – 1977*, Landers DM and Christina RW (Eds). Human Kinetics, Champaign, Illinois, USA, pp. 106–129

Landers DM (1980) The arousal–performance relationship revisited. *Res Quart Exer Sport* **51**: 77–90

Lee DN and Young DS (1985) Visual timing of interceptive action. In: *Brain mechanisms and spatial vision*, Ingle D, Jeannerod M and Lee DN (Eds). Nijhoff, Dordrecht, Holland, pp. 1–30

Lee DN, Lishman JR and Thompson JA (1984) Regulation of gait in long jumping. *J Exp Psych: Human Perception and Performance* **81**: 448–459

Lee TD and Magill RA (1983) The locus of contextual interference in motor skill acquisition. *J Exp Psych: Learning, Memory and Cognition* **9**: 730–746

Lenoir N *et al.* (1999) Intercepting moving objects during self-motion. *J Motor Behavior* **31**: 55–67

MacGillivary WW (1980) The contribution of perceptual style to human performance. *Int J Sport Psych* **11**: 132–141

MacNeilage PF (1970) Motor control of serial ordering of speech. *Psych Rev* **77**: 182–196

Magill RA (1993) *Motor learning: concepts and applications, 4th edn.* Brown and Benchmark, Madison, Wisconsin, USA

Masters RSW (2000) Theoretical aspects of implicit learning in sport. *Int J Sport Psych* **31**: 530–541

McGarry T and Franks IM (1997) A horse race between independent processes: Evidence for a phantom point of no return in the preparation of a speeded motor response. *J Exp Psych: Human Perception and Performance* **23**: 1533–1542

McLeod B (1985) Field dependence as a factor in sports with preponderance of open and closed skills. *Perceptual and Motor Skills* **60**: 369–370

McLeod P (1987) Visual reaction time and high-speed ball games. *Perception* **16**: 49–59

McLeod P and Jenkins S (1991) Timing accuracy and decision time in high-speed ball games. *Int J Sport Psych* **22**: 279–295

McMorris T (1986) An investigation into the relationship between cognitive style and decision making in soccer. Unpublished Master's thesis, University of New Brunswick, Canada

McMorris T (1992) Field independence and performance in sport. *Int J Sport Psych* **23**: 14–27

McMorris T (1997) Performance of soccer players on tests of field dependence/independence and soccer-specific decision-making tests. *Perceptual and Motor Skills* **85**: 467–476

McMorris T and Cobb P (1993) Motivation of and field dependence of males and females engaging in team and individual sports. In: *Motivation, emotion and stress*, Nitsch JR and Seiler R (Eds). Academia, Sankt Augustin, pp. 86–90

McMorris T and MacGillivary WW (1988) An investigation into the relationship between field independence and decision making in soccer. In: *Science and football*, Reilly T *et al.* (Eds). Spon, London, UK, pp. 552–557

McMorris T *et al.* (1993) Scores on field independence and performance in snooker. *Perceptual and Motor Skills* **77**: 1151–1154

Miller GA (1956) The magical number seven, plus or minus two: some limits on our capacity for processing information. *Psych Rev* **63**: 81–97

Nacsson J and Schmidt RA (1971) The activity-set hypothesis for warm-up decrement. *J Motor Behavior* **3**: 1–15

Newell KM (1986) Constraints on the development of coordination, In: *Motor development in children: aspects of coordination and control*, Wade MG and Whiting HTA (Eds). Nijhoff, Dordrecht, Holland, pp. 341–360

Nicholls JG (1984) Achievement motivation: conceptions of ability, subjective experience, task choice, and performance. *Psych Rev* **91**: 328–346

Norman DA (1969) *Memory and attention*. Wiley, New York, USA

Osgood CE (1949) The similarity paradox in human learning: A resolution. *Psych Rev* **56**: 132–143

Oxendine JB (1968) *Psychology of motor learning, 1st edn*. Appleton-Century-Crofts, New York, USA

Pargman D (1977) Perceptual cognitive ability as a function of race, sex and academic achievement in college athletes. *Int J Sport Psych* **8**: 79–91

Pargman D, Schreiber LE and Stein F (1974) Field dependence of selected athletic sub-groups. *Med Sci Sports* **6**: 283–286

Pascual-Leone J (1989) An organismic process model of Witkin's Field-Dependence-Independence. In: *Cognitive style and cognitive development*, Globerson T and Zelniker T (Eds). Ablex, Norwood, New Jersey, USA, pp. 36–70

Piaget J (1952) *The origins of intelligence in children*. International Universities Press, New York, USA

Piaget J (1969) *The psychology of the child*. Basic Books, New York, USA

Poulton EC (1957) On prediction in skilled movements. *Psych Bull* **54**: 467–478

Pribram KH and McGuinness D (1975) Arousal, activation, and effort in the control of attention. *Psych Rev* **82**: 116–149

Quesada DC and Schmidt RA (1970) A test of the Adams–Creamer decay hypothesis for the timing of motor responses. *J Motor Behavior* **2**: 273–283

Ripoll H and Latiri I (1997) Effect of expertise on coincident-timing accuracy in a fast ball game. *J Sport Sci* **15**: 573–580

Roberts GC (1984) Towards a new theory of motivation in sport. The role of perceived ability. In: *Psychological foundations of sport*, Silva J and Weinberg B (Eds). Human Kinetics, Champaign, Illinois, USA, pp. 214–229

Salmela JH and Fiorito P (1979) Visual cues in ice hockey goal-tending. *Can J Appl Sport Sci* **4**: 51–59

Sanders AF (1983) Towards a model of stress and human performance. *Acta Psych* **53**: 61–97

Schmidt RA (1975) A schema theory of discrete motor skill learning *Psych Rev* **82**: 225–260

Shea JB and Morgan RL (1979) Contextual interference effects on the acquisition, retention and transfer of a motor skill. *J Exp Psych: Human Learning and Memory* **5**: 179–187

Sherrington CS (1906) *The integrative action of the nervous system*. Yale University Press, New Haven, USA

Singer RN (1968) *Motor Control and human performance, 1st edn.* Macmillan, London, UK

Skinner BF (1953) *Science and human behaviour.* Macmillan, New York, USA

Spence KW (1958) A theory of emotionally based drive and its relation to performance in simple learning situations. *Am Psych* **13**: 131–141

Starkes JL (1987) Skill in field hockey: the nature of the cognitive advantage. *J Sport Psych* **9**: 146–160

Swets JA (1964) Is there a sensory threshold? In: *Signal detection and recognition by human observers*, Swets JA (Ed). Wiley, New York, USA, pp. 122–144

Swets JA and Green DM (1964) Sequential observations by human observers of signals in noise. In: *Signal detection and recognition by human observers*, Swets JA (Ed). Wiley, New York, USA, pp. 221–242

Tenenbaum G *et al.* (1993) The relationship between cognitive characteristics and decision making. *Can J Appl Phys* **18**: 48–62

Thiffault C (1980) Construction et validation d'une mesure de la rapidité de la pensée tactique des jouers de hockey sur glace (The construction and validation of a measure of tactical thought of ice hockey players) In: *Psychology of motor behavior and sport – 1979*, Nadeau C *et al.* (Eds). Human Kinetics, Champaign, Illinois, USA, pp. 643–649

Thorndike EL (1927) The law of effect. *Am J Psych* **29**: 212–222

Treisman AM (1964) Monitoring and storage of irrelevant messages in selective attention. *J Verbal Learning and Verbal Behavior* **3**: 449–459

Trevarthen CB (1968) Two mechanisms of vision in primates. *Psychologische Forschung* **31**: 299–337

Tulving E (1985) How many memory systems are there? *Am Psych* **40**: 385–398

Turvey MT (1992) Ecological foundations of cognition: invariants of perception and action. In: *Cognition: conceptual and methodological issues*, Pick H, Van Den P and Knill D (Eds). American Psychological Association, Washington, DC, USA, pp. 85–117

Turvey MT *et al.* (1981) Ecological laws of perceiving and acting: In reply to Fodor and Pylyshyn (1981). *Cognition* **9**: 237–304

Vygotsky LS (1978) *Mind in society.* Harvard University Press, Cambridge, Massachusetts, USA

Welford AT (1968) *Fundamentals of skill*. Methuen, London, UK

White SA and Duda JL (1994) The relationship of gender, level of sport involvement, and participation motivation to task ands ego orientation. *Int J Sport Psych* 25: 4–18

Williams AM and Davids K (1995) Declarative knowledge in sport: a by-product of experience or a characteristic of expertise? *J Sport Exer Psych* 17: 259–275

Williams AM and Davids K (1998) Visual search strategy, selective attention, and expertise in soccer. *Res Quart Exer Sport* 69: 111–128

Witkin HA (1950) Individual differences in ease of perception of embedded figures. *J Personality* 19: 1–15

Witkin HA and Goodenough DR (1980) *Cognitive style: essence and origins*. International Universities Press, New York, USA

Witkin HA *et al.* (1970) *Group embedded figures test*. Consulting Psychology Press, Palo Alto, California, USA

Witkin HA *et al.* (1971) *Manual for the embedded figures tests*. Consulting Psychologists Press, Palo Alto, California, USA, p. 8

Yerkes RM and Dodson JD (1908) The relation of strength of stimulus to rapidity of habit formation. *J Comp Neurol Psych* 18: 459–482

Index

Acquisition and Performance of Sports Skills T. McMorris
© 2004 John Wiley & Sons, Ltd   ISBNs: 0-470-84994-0 (HB); 0-470-84995-9 (PB)